Mitigation of Cancer Therapy Side-Effects with Light

Mitigation of Cancer Therapy Side-Effects with Light

Raj Nair
Griffith University and Menzies Health Institute Queensland
Gold Coast University Hospital, Queensland Health, Gold Coast, Australia

René-Jean Bensadoun
Responsable de Service, Centre de Haute Energie (CHE), Nice, France

Morgan & Claypool Publishers

ISBN 978-1-6817-4075-1 (ebook)
ISBN 9781643278858 (print)
ISBN 978-1-6817-4203-8 (mobi)

DOI 10.1088/978-1-6817-4075-1

Version: 20161001

IOP Concise Physics
ISSN 2053-2571 (online)
ISSN 2054-7307 (print)

A Morgan & Claypool publication as part of IOP Concise Physics
Published by Morgan & Claypool Publishers, 40 Oak Drive, San Rafael, CA, 94903 USA

IOP Publishing, Temple Circus, Temple Way, Bristol BS1 6HG, UK

To Natsha, Ramil and Anut - Raj Nair

To my loving family - Rene-Jean Bensadoun

Contents

Preface

'Light' from low level laser therapy, through a process called photobiomodulation (PBM), has been in existence in supportive care in cancer, in particular in the management of oral mucositis (OM) in patients undergoing chemotherapy, radiation therapy and haematopoietic stem cell transplantation.

Possible ways in which PBM has an impact on the disease state are through modulation of ulceration, inflammation, oedema, pain, fibrosis, and neurological and muscular injury. PBM parameters for prophylactic and therapeutic use in supportive care for OM, dermatitis, dysphagia, dry mouth, dysgeusia, trismus, necrosis, lymphedema and voice/speech alterations are discussed. For convenience, we have designated sections according to the symptoms and each section describes a literature search, followed by a description of how, when and where to apply PBM for specific symptoms, such as, for example, OM.

Introduction

Humanity has conquered many unfathomable obstacles, and thrives to learn and continuously achieve more, particularly in the field of medicine. The fight against ailments is infinite as we evolve through the different facets of 'ultra'-modernisation with improved cancer diagnosis, care and survivorship.

From cancer diagnosis and through survivorship, disease and treatment-related complications arise and must be dealt with using the utmost care, as often these complications may jeopardise the cancer treatment itself. Avoiding the addition of drugs to control these complications to the already long list of the cancer regimen is the aim of any supportive care clinician. A low level laser, unlike the name indicates, is only a source of 'light', or visible light in the spectrum. Light in this frequency has effects on a cellular level, depending upon the area of application, the depth and the dosage, without producing any heat energy.

This book is an attempt to portray the current status of the supportive care interventions that are possible with photobiomodulation (PBM) using low level laser therapy (LLLT) in patients undergoing cancer treatment for solid tumours, haematological malignancies, and head and neck cancers.

Acknowledgement

This book is made possible from the extensive literature search, study group exercises, consultations with experts, scientific presentations and resultant publications and we wish to acknowledge those innumerable souls who have contributed and worked along with us in the past decades. Naturally, it is beyond the scope of this humble initiative to name all but may we take this opportunity to thank each one of you.

About the authors

Raj Nair

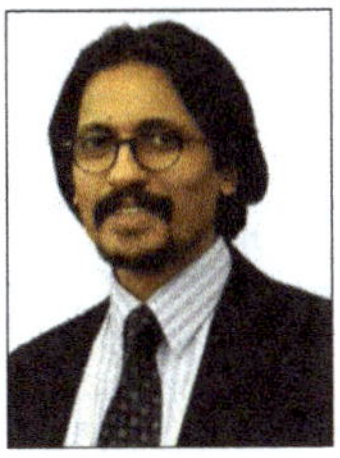

Raj is a Professor of Oral Medicine/Oral Oncology, Acting Deputy Head of School (Research), Higher Degree Research (HDR) Convenor, Discipline Head of Oral Medicine, Oral Pathology and Human Diseases at Griffith University and Oral Oncology Consultant, Department of Haematology and Oncology (Cancer Services), Gold Coast University Hospital (GCUH), Queensland Health, Gold Coast, Australia. He is a member of Cancer Research group of Menzies Health Institute Queensland. Raj is an educator who convenes university courses in the discipline of oral medicine, oral pathology, and internal medicine and contributes to the education of specialist trainees and nurses at the hospital. He is Honorary Associate Professor at the University of Queensland, Brisbane, Australia.

He has received his oral medicine/oncology clinical training as a fellow at Harvard and affiliated hospitals, USA and from the University of London, UK and research scholarship recipient, Centre for Blood Disorders, Harvard Medical School. He obtained his PhD from the University of Hong Kong in 1996. He was awarded membership in the special stream of Oral Medicine by the Royal Australasian College of Dental Surgeons (RACDS) in 2008.

He is an internationally renowned clinician and researcher in the fields of oral medicine, oral oncology and orofacial supportive care and the management of cancer patients on chemotherapy, radiation therapy, and hematopoietic stem cell transplantation. He has over 100 publications and book chapter contributions. Internationally, he has served as an invited speaker and presenter of numerous scientific research papers in the past two decades. His current research projects include microbiome and cancer and international multi-centre studies on photobiomodulation (PBM) in cancer-therapy induced complications and burden of illness especially oral mucositis and other complications amongst cancer patients in partnership with universities in the USA and Europe.

He is a member of International Society of Oral Oncology (ISOO), Multinational Association of Supportive Care in Cancer (MASCC), American Academy of Oral Medicine, Harvard Club of Australia and International Association for Dental Research. He serves as invited consultant at international consensus bodies such as World Workshop in Oral Medicine, World Workshop in Oral Health and Diseases in AIDS. He was a director-councillor of the RACDS and currently director board member of ISOO and IADR oral medicine/pathology section and founding board member of International Group in Light in Oncology-Barcelona (iGLOB). He is chair of PBM in cancer working group and chair of the PBM study group/mucositis study group of MASCC.

René-Jean Bensadoun

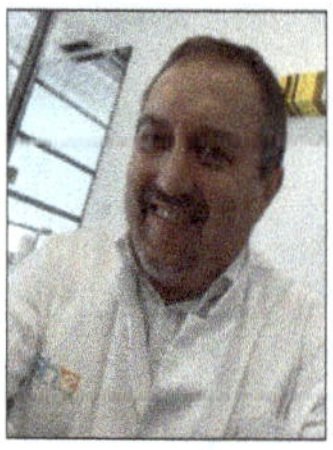

Professor René-Jean Bensadoun is a Radiation Oncologist and Professor of Oncology-Radiotherapy. He was Head of Radiotherapy Department at the Centre Antoine Lacassagne in Nice (2006–2008), and Head of the Department of Radiotherapy at the University Hospital of Poitiers, Regional Cancer Pole, from 2008 to 2014. He currently heads the Nice High Energy Centre (private structure of Radiotherapy and Supportive Care).

His special interests are in the field of aerodigestive tract cancers and in the dosimetry of photobiomodulation using low level light in supportive care in cancer and cancer therapy complications, since the early 1980's. He was involved in several clinical trials and meta-analysis position articles in the field of radiation and chemotherapy-induced oral mucositis.

Professor Bensadoun has published over 220 articles in peer-reviewed journals, 69 as first or last author, and authored two books published in the US on the use of low-energy laser in cancer. His key publication with Professor Bjordal has led to the World Association of Laser Therapy (WALT) guidelines for the use of Photobiomodulation in Oncology. He is very active in organizing theoretical and practical courses in Photobiomodulation in France with Dr Pelletier of the European LED Academy.

He is currently the scientific secretary of World Association for Laser Therapy (WALT), a Member of the Board of the French Society of Oncology Neck-Facial, Groupe Oncologie Radiotherapie Tête et Cou (GORTEC), AFSOS, LED Academy, and Multinational Association for Supportive Care in Cancer (MASCC).

Other contributing authors

Judith A E M Zecha, Department of Oral and Maxillofacial Surgery Academic Medical Center, University of Amsterdam, Meibergdreef 9 1105 AZ, Amsterdam, The Netherlands

Judith E Raber-Durlacher, Department of Oral and Maxillofacial Surgery, Academic Medical Center Amsterdam, Department of Medical Dental Interaction and Department of Periodontology, Academic Centre for Dentistry, Amsterdam (ACTA), University of Amsterdam and VU University, Amsterdam, The Netherlands; PO Box 22660 1100 DD, Amsterdam, The Netherlands

Joel B Epstein, Samuel Oschin Comprehensive Cancer Institute, Cedars-Sinai Medical Center, Los Angeles, CA 90048,USA; Division of Otolaryngology and Head and Neck Surgery, City of Hope, Duarte, CA 91010, USA

James Carrol, CEO, Thorlaser, UK

Mitigation of Cancer Therapy Side-Effects with Light

Raj Nair and René-Jean Bensadoun

Section 1. Photobiomodulation and low level laser therapy

LLLT/PBM has been consistently shown in laboratory studies to have distinct biological effects, and has a dose-dependent mechanism of action at the cellular level. Since the introduction of LLLT/PBM in 1967, over 400 randomized, double-blind (some placebo-controlled) clinical trials have been published for multiple applications. The first clinical application of LLLT/PBM was for the enhancement of wound healing. A meta-analysis including animal and human studies concluded that LLLT/PBM was an effective tool for accelerating wound repair and tissue regeneration. It has been shown that LLLT/PBM influences different phases of wound healing including: (i) the inflammatory phase, in which immune cells migrate to the site of tissue injury; (ii) the proliferative phase, which includes stimulation of fibroblasts and macrophages as well as other repair components; and (iii) the remodelling phase, consisting of collagen deposition and rebuilding of the extra-cellular matrix at the wound site.

Although the complex biological mechanisms underlying the therapeutic effects of LLLT/PBM have not been completely elucidated and may vary among different cell types and tissue states (healthy versus stressed or hypoxic), laboratory and clinical studies suggest that LLLT/PBM significantly reduces inflammation and prevents fibrosis. Moreover, LLLT/PBM, when delivered appropriately, reduces pain and improves optimal function of the whole organism. In addition, *in vivo* studies show that LLLT/PBM is neuroprotective and may benefit neurodegenerative diseases and neurotrauma.

Current data suggest that LLLT/PBM acts predominantly on cytochrome c oxidase (CcO) in the mitochondrial respiratory chain by facilitating electron transport resulting in an increased transmembrane proton gradient that drives adenosine triphosphate (ATP) production. ATP is the universal energy source in living cells and is essential for all biological reactions; even a small increase in ATP levels can enhance the bioavailability to power the functions of cellular metabolism. In addition, the absorption of red or near-infrared (NIR) light may cause a short, transient burst of reactive oxygen species (ROS) that are followed by an adaptive reduction in oxidative stress.

doi:10.1088/978-1-6817-4075-1ch1

A low concentration of ROS activates many cellular processes, since ROS activates transcription factors including nuclear factor kappa B (NF-κB), resulting in the upregulation of stimulatory and protective genes. These genes generate growth factors belonging to the fibroblast growth factor family, cytokines, and chemokines that are involved in tissue repair.

In hypoxic or otherwise stressed cells, mitochondria produce nitric oxide (mtNO), which binds to CcO and displaces oxygen. This binding results in inhibition of cellular respiration, decreased ATP production and increased oxidative stress (a state that develops when the levels of ROS exceed the defence mechanisms), leading to the activation of intracellular signalling pathways, including several transcription factors. These include the redox factor-1 (Ref-1), activator protein-1 (AP-1), NF-κB, p53, activating transcription factor/cAMP-response element-binding protein (ATF/CREB), hypoxia-inducible factor (HIF)-1 and HIF-like factor. These transcription factors induce down-stream production of both inflammatory mediators, such as tumour necrosis factor-alpha (TNF-α), Interleukin (IL)-1 and IL-6, cyclo-oxygenase (COX)-2 and prostaglandin E2 (PGE-2), and anti-inflammatory mediators (TGF-β, IL10). There is evidence suggesting that when LLLT/PBM is administered with appropriate parameters to stressed cells, NO is dissociated from its competitive binding to CcO, ATP production is increased, and the balance between pro- and antioxidant mediators is restored, resulting in a reduction of oxidative stress. For example, LLLT/PBM has been shown to attenuate the production of ROS by human neutrophils. LLLT/PBM reduced ROS in an animal model of traumatic tissue injury; whereas in a model of acute lung inflammation LLLT/PBM was found to reduce the generation of TNF-α and to increase IL-10, an anti-inflammatory cytokine. In addition, NO is a potent vasodilator and can increase the blood-supply to the illuminated tissue. LLLT-mediated vascular regulation increases tissue oxygenation and also allows for greater traffic of immune cells. These two effects may contribute to the promotion of wound repair and regeneration.

Analgesic effects are probably induced by additional mechanisms rather than by the increased ATP/reduced oxidative stress model. LLLT/PBM with a relatively high power density (>300 (milliwatts) mW cm^{-2}), when absorbed by nociceptors, has an inhibitory effect on A and C neuronal pain fibres. This slows the neural conduction velocity, reduces amplitude of compound action potentials and suppresses neurogenic inflammation.

Virtually all conditions modulated by LLLT/PBM (e.g. ulceration, inflammation, oedema, pain, fibrosis, neurological and muscular injury) are thought to be involved in the pathogenesis of (chemo)radiotherapy ((C)RT)-induced complications in patients treated for head and neck cancer (HNC). For example, in an animal model of oral mucositis (OM) it was demonstrated that LLLT/PBM decreased COX-2 expression and decreased the number of neutrophils in the inflammatory infiltrate. Moreover, in the chronic sequelae of (C)RT an excessive fibroblastic response is hypothesized to be related to acute oxidative injury, with resulting cell damage, ischemia, and an ongoing inflammatory response resulting in fibrosis. The critical difference between normal wound healing and fibrosis development appears to be that in fibrosis, signalling pathways escape normal cellular regulation. The reduction of fibrosis could be mediated by the beneficial effects of LLLT/PBM on the oxidant/antioxidant balance down-regulation of the profibrotic transforming growth factor-beta (TGF-β) and inhibition of excessive fibroblast proliferation.

The efficacy of LLLT/PBM in both acute and chronic conditions and affected tissues has been shown to be promising in the majority of studies, although not all have yielded positive outcomes. These divergent results may be attributed to factors including dosimetry. It has been observed that increasing the overall dose of LLLT/PBM may have a counter-productive effect compared to the benefit obtained with lower doses

LLLT/PBM parameters

The LLLT/PBM parameters (summarized in table 1.1) are usually within the red and NIR wavelength range of 600–1000 nanometres (nm), with a power density of between 5–150 mW cm^{-2} and are typically applied for 30–60 s per point. The therapeutic effect is typically dictated by the energy density measured in joules (J) cm^{-2}. Experimental evidence can be found in the literature for parameters as widely divergent as 0.1–12 J cm^{-2}. Laser systems used include helium–neon (HeNe), gallium–aluminium (GaAl), neodymium-doped yttrium–aluminium–garnet (Nd: YAG), gallium–aluminium–arsenide (GaAlAs) diode, indium–gallium–aluminium–phosphorus (InGaAlP), and non-thermal, non-ablative carbon dioxide (CO_2) lasers.

The PBM effects on the exposed tissues depend upon the cell type, redox state of the cell, irradiation parameters (wavelength, power density) and time of exposure. A biphasic dose response has been shown in several studies, which underlines that there are optimal irradiation and dose parameters, although these will vary depending upon the depth of the pathology below the mucosal or skin surface. One must remember that doses lower than the optimal value may have a reduced effect, while doses higher than optimal can have negative therapeutic outcomes.

For LLLT/PBM to be effective, the irradiation parameters—including the energy delivered, power density, pulse structure, delivery to the appropriate anatomical location, and appropriate treatment timing and repetition—need to be within the biostimulatory dose windows. This has been shown by studies which demonstrate negative effects where dose depends on energy dose level alone. Titrating adequate doses and defining the other required laser parameters according to evidence gathered in a systematic way for each indication is a prerequisite for the successful use of this technique. Without standardization in beam measurement, dose calculation, and the correct reporting of these parameters, studies will not be reproducible, and outcomes will not be consistent. A common misconception is that wavelength and energy (in J) or energy density (J cm^{-2}) are all that is necessary in order to replicate a successful treatment, and that it does not matter what the original power, power density, and duration of application were.

Table 1.1. LLLT parameters.

Category	Parameter	Unit	Explanation
Irradiation parameters	Wavelength	Nanometre (nm)	Light is packets of electromagnetic energy called photons that sometimes behave like particles but also have a wave-like property. Wavelength determines which chromophores will absorb the light. Light is visible in the 400–700 nm range. The energy of each photon is greater at short wavelengths than longer wavelengths; e.g. red light is ~2 electronvolts (eV) per photon and blue light is ~3 eV.
	Power	Watt (W)	The number of photons per second. The higher the power the more photons emitted every second.
	Beam area	Centimetre squared (cm^2)	The surface area of the beam on the patient. Also known as spot size. This is not always easy to determine because laser beams are usually more intense in the middle then fade towards the edge (Gaussian distribution) so it is hard to define where the exact edge of the beam is without special instruments. Many research authors do not report this parameter, let alone report it correctly.
	Aperture size	Centimetre squared (cm^2)	The area of the light source tip. This is not necessarily identical to the beam area. The difference between the aperture size and beam area will be determined by the beam divergence and distance of the light source tip from the tissue.
	Irradiance (power density, or intensity)	Watts per centimetre squared ($W\ cm^{-2}$)	Power (W) ÷ beam area (cm^2). More irradiance could allow less treatment time, however many studies have shown that if the irradiance is too high, treatment can be less effective even if the same total dose is delivered. The treatment guidelines suggest the safe and effective irradiance ranges.

	(Radiant) Energy	Joules (J)	Power (W) × time (s). More power could mean less treatment time however many studies have shown that too much power is less effective even if the same total energy is delivered. The treatment guidelines suggest the safe and effective energy ranges.
	Time	Second (s)	How long each treatment is applied at each location.
	Dosage (fluence or energy density)	Joules per centimetre squared ($J\ cm^{-2}$)	Energy (J) ÷ beam area (cm^2), or power (W) ÷ beam area (cm^2) × time (s). Different outcomes can be obtained if the total dosage is delivered with high energy and short time or low energy and long time.
	Operating mode	Continuous wave (CW), pulsed	The continuity of the production of the output beam may be continuous or pulsed. There are several types of pulsed beam.
	Pulse structure	Second(s)	The durations of the pulse being on or off.
Treatment parameters	Physical relationship to the organ		Applicable when there is more than one way to approach the organ. For example, intra-oral device versus extra-oral device.
	Timing		Time of the treatment session relative to the cancer treatment.
	Treatment schedule		The frequency of treatments per day/week and the total number of treatments.
	Anatomical location		The anatomical site that was exposed to the light beam. If multiple locations were treated, all need to be described.

Table 1.1 provides a checklist to help researchers understand and report all the necessary parameters for a reproducible scientific study. In addition, it is not uncommon to find discrepancies between the specifications provided by a device manufacturer and the actual performance of the device. Thus, device maintenance, including power measurements, should be carried out regularly during research trials and also in clinical practice.

Section 2. Dermatitis

Radiation dermatitis occurs in the majority of patients with loco-regionally advanced HNC treated with RT.

The pathobiology of acute radiation dermatitis is complex and partially overlaps that of OM. Irradiation of the skin leads to direct tissue injury and inflammatory cell recruitment, leading to damage to epidermal basal cells, endothelial cells and vascular components. Radiation-induced generation of free radicals causing DNA injury and release of inflammatory cytokines (in particular IL-1 and IL-6) lead to clinical changes such as erythema, oedema and possible ulceration. Late RT-induced changes in the skin are characterized by the disappearance of follicular structures, an increase in collagen and damage to elastic fibres in the dermis, and a fragile epidermal covering. TGF-β is considered to play a central role in mediating RT-induced tissue fibrosis.

The total radiation dose, dose per fraction, overall treatment time, beam type and energy, surface area of the skin exposed to radiation, use of combined CRT with or without targeted therapies, and individual risk factors, all contribute to the severity of skin reactions. The severity of acute reactions has been shown to predict late effects. Radiation dermatitis impacts adversely on cosmesis and function, particularly in patients with secondarily infected irradiated skin, and reduces quality of life (QoL).

Table 1.2. Radiation dermatitis treatment parameters.

Radiation dermatitis	*Prophylactic*: Start daily PBM treatment at the initiation of RT, or with a grade 1 radiation dermatitis *Therapeutic*: Continue treatment at least 3 times a week until symptoms improve	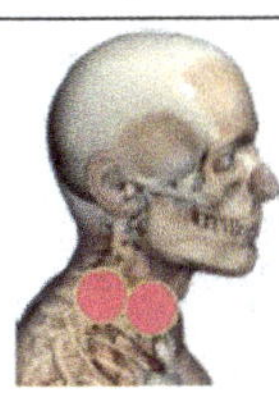	*Extra-oral*: Red laser diode cluster, 630–680 nm, 20–150 mW cm^{-2} or Mixed red and IR LED cluster 20–80 mW cm^{-2}	*Extra-oral*: *Prophylactic*: 2 J cm^{-2} for laser diode panel. 3 J cm^{-2} for extra oral LED cluster *Therapeutic*: At least 4 J cm^{-2}	*Extra-oral*: Cutaneous surfaces on the radiation field where dermatitis is anticipated (often erythematous after RT)

Patients with squamous cell carcinoma (SCC) of the head and neck treated with an epidermal growth factor receptor (EGFR)-inhibitor may develop an acneiform skin rash in addition to radiation dermatitis.

Based on the effects of LLLT/PBM on the epidermis and dermis (reduced inflammation and improved wound healing), and on the shared similarities in pathobiology with OM, it seems reasonable to assume that LLLT/PBM may reduce the severity and/or prevalence of radiation dermatitis. Multi-wavelength LLLT/PBM ameliorated the development of late radiation damage to the skin in an animal model. LED treatment immediately after intensity modulated RT (IMRT) reduced the incidence of radiation dermatitis in patients with breast cancer, but these results could not be reproduced, although important parameters such as irradiation time and size of area treated were not reported. Promising results have been reported for LLLT laser treatment at a NIR wavelength (970 nm) in patients with EGFR inhibitor-induced facial rash.

Section 3. Lymphedema

Lymphedema as a consequence of cancer treatment is apparent in breast cancer and HNC. In the case of HNC, it has been one of the neglected late effects, although these complications may be reduced with IMRT. In HNC patients, lymphedema may develop externally, on the face and neck, and/or internally involving the larynx and pharynx. External lymphedema may have a profound effect on body image, whereas internal lymphedema may interfere with breathing, contribute to dysphagia and trismus, and may affect speech.

Lymphedema has been reported in high numbers in HNC, for example, a single centre study on 81 HNC patients reported 75% incidence with 10% external, 39% internal and 51% experiencing both types of lymphedema. Individuals with pharyngeal carcinoma were at highest risk. Chronic lymphedema that develops later (2–6 months after) may resolve spontaneously in some patients, but not in all.

The pathobiology of lymphedema consists of an initiation where disruption of lymphatic structures occurs by surgery or RT, resulting in the accumulation of lymph fluid in the interstitial tissues. This leads to infiltration of inflammatory cells

Table 1.3. Head and neck lymphedema treatment parameters.

Head and neck lymphedema	*Therapeutic*: Continue treatment at least 2 or 3 times a week until symptoms improve	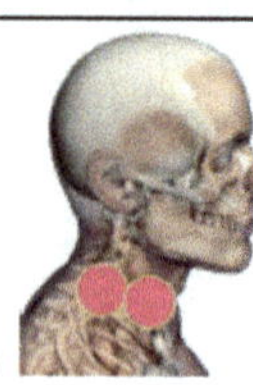	*Extra-oral*: IR laser diodes or LED cluster 750–830 nm 20–80 mW cm^{-2}	*Extra-oral*: 3 J cm^2 laser diodes or LED cluster	*Extra-oral*: Treat edematous area over the neck or surgical site if any, also targeting regional lymphatic chain

and, because of the lymphatic dysfunction, cytokines and chemokines remain in the tissue and recruit additional inflammatory cells from the circulation. This ongoing vicious inflammatory response results in additional soft tissue damage and fibrosis, which further adversely affects lymphatic function.

In breast cancer patients, LLLT has been identified as a potential treatment for post-mastectomy lymphedema, as it stimulates lymphangiogenesis, enhances lymphatic motility, and reduces lymphostatic fibrosis. Patients received additional benefits from LLLT/PBM when used in conjunction with standard lymphedema treatment. Systematic reviews found evidence suggesting that LLLT/PBM reduced limb volume in patients with lymphedema following treatment for breast cancer. Future research is needed comparing LLLT/PBM to standard practices to establish the duration of laser application, number of treatment sessions, energy settings, power density and dose, using longer follow-up.

Section 4. Mucositis

OM affects virtually all patients undergoing CRT for advanced HNC, and the majority of haematopoietic stem cell transplantation (HSCT) and high dose CT regimens. Clinically, the manifestations of OM form a continuum, with erythematous mucosal changes when mild and ulcerative lesions that expose the submucosa in its severe form. Its detrimental effects on QoL and functional status are significant and often interfere with the cancer treatment regimen, both on the patient level and in terms of cost.

The current understanding of OM is largely based on animal models, which have shown the multifactorial nature of the condition and have implicated a cascade of interrelated events in multiple tissue regions. These observations combine into the five-phase model of OM, based on the sequence of events following cytotoxic treatment. The formation of excessive ROS and activation of NF-κB are the key factors in its pathobiology. Subsequent studies have implicated microvascular injury, the formation of proinflammatory cytokines, host–microbiome interactions and extracellular matrix alterations in OM pathogenesis. In addition, EGFR inhibitors and tyrosine kinase receptor inhibitors (TKIs) administered as single drug or combined with CRT may enhance OM or cause additional symptoms. Effective management options for OM are still scarce, and pain control is often inadequate.

A Cochrane meta-analysis and a systematic review and meta-analysis from 2011 on 11 randomised control trials (RCTs) in HNC patients treated with CT and/or RT concluded that there was consistent evidence that LLLT/PBM applied with doses of 1–6 J per point reduced OM prevalence, severity and duration, and associated pain. Another meta-analysis including RCTs in various cancer treatment settings showed that LLLT/PBM reduced OM risk and decreased its severity and duration. The efficacy appeared to be similar for red (630–670 nm) and NIR (780–830 nm) light, although the optimal doses seemed to vary between

Table 1.4. Mucositis treatment parameters

Complication	Treatment protocol	Treatment area	PBM device characteristics and application	Therapeutic PBM dose	Optional target tissues
Oral Mucositis	*Prophylactic*: *Chemotherapy*: Protocols vary. Start PBM treatment at first day of CT or prior to therapy and continue during all courses of chemotherapy *Radiotherapy*: Start PBM treatment the first day of RT or prior to RT and continue during all days of RT (no requirement regarding the timing of PBM sessions, before or after RT session) *Therapeutic*: Continue treatment at least 3 times a week until symptoms improve Daily treatment is recommended in case of severe mucositis	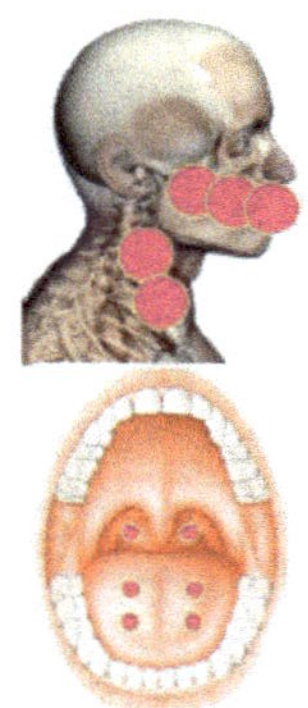	*Extra-oral*: IR LED cluster or mixed red and IR LED cluster 20–80 mW cm^{-2} *Intra-oral*: 630–830 nm 20–80 mW	*Extra-oral*: 3 J cm^{-2} IR LED cluster *Intra-oral*: *Prophylactic*: 2 J per point *Therapeutic*: 4 J per point until the whole area involved is covered (2 J for prophylactic use)	*Extra-oral*: Lips, cutaneous surface corresponding to the buccal mucosae, bilateral cervical lymphatic chain *Intra-oral*: *Prophylactic*: treat each of the at risk mucosal surfaces *Therapeutic*: sites vary, depending upon the site of mucositis

these wavelengths. Similarly, a systematic review and meta-analysis including 18 RCTs reported that prophylactic LLLT/PBM reduced severe OM and associated pain in patients treated for HNC or undergoing HSCT. The Clinical Practice Guidelines of the Multinational Association of Supportive Care in Cancer and International Society for Oral Oncology (MASCC/ISOO) Mucositis Study Group found evidence for LLLT/PBM prevention of OM in patients undergoing HSCT, and patients treated with RT for HNC. Evidence was derived from high quality studies using specific LLLT/PBM parameters and the study group noted that there remains a need to identify optimal LLLT/PBM parameters, including energy density, ideal timing of laser application, variations in cancer type and cancer treatment regimens.

Based on this evidence and on our experience, we propose the following regimen for the management of OM (and mucositis affecting the oropharynx): a wavelength of 633–685 nm or 780–830 nm; a power output of between 10 and 150 mW; an energy density of 2–3 J cm^{-2} and no more than 6 J cm^{-2} on the tissue surface treated; a frequency of 2–3 times a week up to daily; and successive applications on single spots on a lesion rather than a scanning motion over the entire lesion. Extra-orally administered LLLT/PBM may be effective for the management of OM of the buccal mucosa, vestibule and inner epithelial surfaces of the lips. This could be applied in combination with an intra-oral device (see table 1.4).

Section 5. Salivary gland—hyposalivation

Another significant complication of RT to the head and neck region is hyposalivation, and its related complaint of xerostomia (subjective oral dryness). For all head and neck radiation regimens pooled, the weighted prevalence of xerostomia was found to be 6% before treatment, 93% during irradiation, and a slightly lower prevalence from one month to more than two years post-treatment. Saliva plays an important role in maintaining mucosal integrity, promoting oral wound healing, taste perception, formation of food bolus, initiation of food ingestion, swallowing and speech. Alterations in the oral microbiota, reduced oral clearance, changes in salival composition such as decreased buffer capacity, pH, immunoglobulin concentrations, defensins and dietary changes may increase the risk for mucosal infections and rapidly progressing dental demineralization and caries. A substantial decrease in salivary function has a significant impact on QoL, and results in an increased burden of long-term oral health care.

Irradiation of the salivary glands results in loss of gland function, beginning early in the course of RT and has been shown to induce apoptosis in parotid glands in a dose-dependent manner. There can be a modest improvement in xerostomia a few months after RT suggesting that an adaptation or compensatory function of non-irradiated salivary glands or a recovery of some of the function occurs. However, most patients have persisting oral dryness for the rest of their life, even when 3D conformal RT is used. With IMRT preserving more of the major salivary

Table 1.5. Hyposalivation treatment parameters.

Hyposalivation and xerostomia	*Prophylactic:* *Radiotherapy*: Start PBM treatment the first day of RT and continue daily with radiation (no requirement regarding the timing of PBM sessions, before or after RT session)	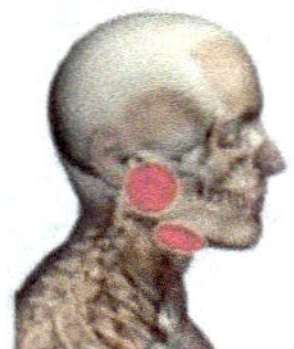 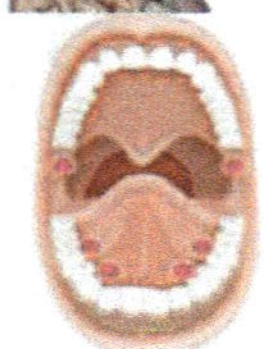	*Extra-oral*: IR laser diodes or LED cluster 750–830 nm 20–80 mW cm^{-2} *Intra-oral*: 630–680 nm 20–150 mW	*Extra-oral*: *Prophylactic*: 3 J cm^{-2} laser diodes or LED cluster *Intra-oral*: *Prophylactic*: 3 J cm^{-2} per point	*Extra-oral*: Major salivary glands, bilaterally (parotid, sublingual and submandibular) *Intra-oral*: Total of 6 points (3 each side) targeting major salivary glands and minor salivary glands (on vestibular side, in the rear of salivary ducts)

glands, long-term oral dryness may be reduced, but a significant proportion of patients may still experience xerostomia.

The literature on LLLT/PBM for the management of hyposalivation is limited. In a study involving a variety of non-cancer patients with xerostomia, LLLT/PBM was applied daily: extra-orally to the parotid and submandibular glands and intra-orally on the sublingual glands. A gradual increase in the stimulated salivary flow was found after LLLT/PBM as compared to controls and similar reports have been documented from non-cancer patients with xerostomia. Animal studies have shown an increase in the number of ductal epithelial cell mitoses, and protein synthesis in submandibular glands following LLLT/PBM. Similarly, there are reports of increased salivary flow rate and amylase activity in rat parotid glands. LLLT/PBM given concurrently with RT could prevent hyposalivation and xerostomia and had an impact on the composition of saliva. Less severe xerostomia was also reported following prophylactic LLLT/PBM in HSCT recipients and in a small RCT in HNC patients treated with RT, and increased salivary flow was observed in LLLT/PBM-treated patients when compared to controls.

These results point to the application of LLLT/PBM for the prevention of hyposalivation and xerostomia; potentially LLLT may also show efficacy for the treatment of hyposalivation when there is any residual function following current RT modalities (the parameters are suggested in table 1.5).

Section 6. Dysphagia

Dysphagia and odynophagia (painful swallowing) are common in HNC patients, particularly in those suffering from oral, oropharyngeal, laryngeal and oesophageal cancers, and those treated with RT or CRT. Dysphagia can be acute or chronic, due to anatomical, mechanical or neurological changes, affecting any structure from the lips to the gastric cardia. Around 60% of patients are reported to have dysphagia following CRT, of which 45% had severe dysphagia at a median of 17 months post-treatment. It has been observed that chronic dysphagia is unlikely to resolve over time.

Dysphagia associated with CRT has a complex pathogenesis, involving acute inflammation, oedema, and fibrosis, with neurological and structural alterations and muscular injury resulting in generalized weakness and a lack of muscle coordination while swallowing. Excessive fibrosis results in a loss of elasticity that may contribute to chronic dysphagia. Furthermore, hyposalivation may contribute to dysphagia following CRT. Duration of total parenteral nutrition (TPN) or nasogastric tube feeding, and resultant reduced swallowing, may affect the ability to return to a safe, normal oral intake and the subsequent inactivity may lead to atrophy of the muscles aiding in the process of swallowing. Dysphagia negatively affects QoL and may predispose sufferers to aspiration and life-threatening pulmonary complications.

Table 1.6. Dysphagia treatment parameters.

Dysphagia	*Prophylactic*: *Radiotherapy*: Start treatment the first day of RT and continue all days of radiation (no requirement regarding the timing of laser sessions, before or after radiation session) *Therapeutic*: Continue treatment at least 3 times a week until symptoms improve	*Extra-oral*: Lateral and ventral pharynx and larynx *Intraoral*: Soft palate, oropharynx	*Extra-oral*: IR laser diodes or LED cluster 750–830 nm 20–80 mW cm^{-2} *Intra-oral*: 630–680 nm 20–150 mW	*Extra-oral*: *Prophylactic*: 3 J cm^{-2} laser diodes or LED cluster *Intra-oral*: *Prophylactic*: 3 J per point	*Extra-oral*: Midline neck and lateral neck anterior to sternocleidomastoid muscle *Intra-oral*: Bilaterally, four points to soft palate and onto oropharynx

IMRT has emerged as an effective technique to deliver the full radiation dose to the tumour and regions at risk, while reducing the exposure of surrounding healthy tissues. Identified dysphagia and aspiration risk structures (DARS) are susceptible to damage during IMRT. In particular, damage to the tongue base, pharyngeal constrictors, the larynx, and the autonomic neural plexus was found to be crucial in the development of post-RT dysphagia. Studies confirmed that reducing the radiation dose to DARS decreases the dysphagia risk, but dysphagia remains a significant clinical problem.

The potential role of LLLT/PBM in the prevention and treatment of dysphagia requires further investigation. One study reported a lower incidence of severe OM and mucositis affecting the throat (contributing to acute dysphagia) when six predetermined oral sites were exposed to LLLT/PBM prior to and during RT. In this study, dysphagia was scored indirectly by assessing the need for TPN. Given the ability of LLLT/PBM to prevent and ameliorate inflammation and pain associated with OM, and the potential to control exuberant fibrosis, LLLT/PBM delivered to the DARSs may have a potential role in the management of acute and chronic dysphagia. The parameters for LLLT/PBM for dysphagia are suggested in table 1.6.

Section 7. Dysgeusia

Altered taste (dysgeusia) is complex and includes difficulties with smell and touch resulting in reduced food interest, affecting appetite and QoL. Taste is one of the five senses and interacts with smell, touch and other physiological cues to affect the wider perception of flavour. Taste function is the perception derived when food molecules stimulate the taste receptors of the tongue, the soft palate and the oropharyngeal region to perceive basic taste qualities (sweet, sour, salty, bitter and umami), measured via standardized methods.

The prevalence of dysgeusia is estimated to be 66.5% following RT alone, and 76.0% after CRT; approximately 15% of patients continued to experience dysgeusia after treatment and it is known that the severity of taste alterations assessed by patients was correlated with the cumulative RT dose.

Table 1.7. Dysgeusia treatment parameters.

Dysgeusia	*Therapeutic*: Continue treatment from the day the patient complains of taste alterations, at least 2 or 3 times a week until symptoms improve	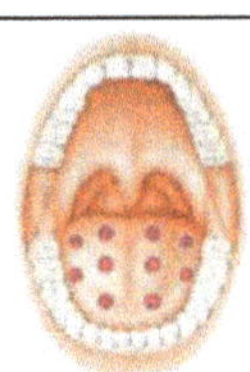	*Intra-oral*: 630–680 nm 20–150 mW	*Intra-oral*: Dorsal and lateral tongue at 3 J cm^{-2}	*Intra-oral*: A total of ten points on the dorsum of the tongue

The mechanisms of dysgeusia during cancer therapy are not well understood. However, it is believed that CT and RT cause dysgeusia by destroying rapidly dividing taste bud cells and olfactory receptor cells. Direct neurologic toxicity may also be involved, as taste recovery lags behind epithelial recovery and may continue indefinitely. Hyposalivation may also make a significant contribution. The presence of the anterior part of the tongue in the radiation field may be predictive for taste disturbances.

Altered taste significantly affects overall QoL and may lead to energy and nutrient deficiencies and related complications and weight loss. Management options to decrease the prevalence and severity of taste problems are inadequate.

A pilot study reported that LLLT/PBM administered to taste buds may ameliorate psychogenic/neurological burning mouth symptoms including taste alterations but, to our knowledge, there are no published studies on LLLT/PBM for the management of taste problems in cancer patients. Hence, we feel that studies on the efficacy of LLLT/PBM for the management of dysgeusia in patients treated for HNC should be performed and the proposed potential LLLT/PBM parameters are provided in table 1.7.

Section 8. Voice alterations

Voice and speech are important communication tools and form part of a person's identity and personality. Voice quality mainly depends on the movement and characteristics of the vocal cords, and speech on the resonance characteristics of the vocal tract. Speech is based on the volitional coordinated movements of the articulator structures and can be affected by any alteration in muscle or tissue properties of these structures. Although voice and speech dysfunctions significantly affect QoL, these complications have received little attention and are likely under-reported in efforts to preserve organ function after cancer therapy.

Currently, there is insufficient information on the prevalence of speech and voice dysfunction in advanced HNC patients treated with CRT. Prospective studies are needed, including baseline measurements and standardized multi-dimensional assessment of functional aspects of voice and speech.

The aetiology of voice and speech problems resembles that of dysphagia and may include neuromuscular weakness as a result of tumour invasion. CRT-induced voice and/or speech dysfunction can result from mucositis of the soft palate and laryngeal soft tissues, fibrosis or vocal fold atrophy, oedema and atrophy of laryngeal and pharyngeal tissues and altered saliva or hyposalivation.

IMRT, designed to spare anatomical structures that are involved with voice and/or speech functions, may well prevent long-term functional impairment and aid early speech rehabilitation.

We are not aware of any studies on the effect of LLLT/PBM on the quality of speech and voice in HNC patients, but LLLT/PBM may preserve function of the anatomical structures involved directly, and could have indirect benefits by decreasing the incidence of hyposalivation.

Table 1.8. Voice alteration treatment parameters.

Voice/speech alterations (due to local inflammation)	*Therapeutic*: Continue treatment from the day patient complains of difficulty speaking, at least 2 or 3 times a week even if symptoms are not improving dramatically	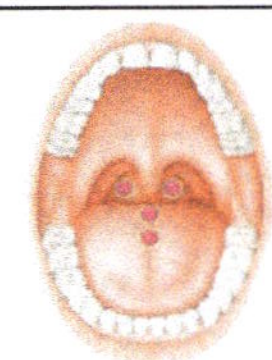	*Intra-oral*: 780–830 nm 50–200 mW	*Intra-oral*: 3 J cm^{-2} per point *Extra-oral*: on larynx area, wavelength 750–830 nm IR laser diodes or LED cluster 20–80 mW/cm^2	*Intra-oral*: Towards the anterior oropharynx over the dorsum of tongue (avoid gag reflex, do not touch any soft tissues including dorsal tongue). Patient may gently close the mouth during the procedure to reduce gag reflex

Section 9. Trismus

Trismus is a restriction or reduced opening of the jaws, due to local infection, tissue fibrosis, pain upon mouth opening, tonic contraction of the muscles of mastication, or a tumour. Trismus has been defined variously as a mouth opening of less than 40 or less than 20 mm, whereas less restrictive classifications also have been used.

The weighted prevalence of trismus is estimated to be 25% following conventional RT, 5% following IMRT and 31% for CRT. Patients may have limitations in jaw opening associated with tumour invasion of the masticatory muscles or the temporomandibular joint, or may develop trismus following RT to these structures. Cumulative radiation doses above 60 Gy are most likely to cause trismus, but the inclusion of the lateral pterygoid muscles in the high dose fields appears to be the most decisive factor. Trismus can be an acute symptom during treatment/RT and typically develops 3–6 months post RT, and frequently becomes a lifelong problem.

Studies have demonstrated that fibrosis is an important initial event in RT-induced trismus. Additionally, there may be scar tissue from surgery, nerve damage, or a combination of these factors. Mandibular hypomobility ultimately results in muscle contraction and potentially temporomandibular joint dysfunction.

Trismus and orofacial pain interfering with function may have significant health implications including reduced nutritional intake, difficulty speaking, compromised oral health and poor QoL. Aside from avoiding RT to the masticatory structures, early interventions are indicated to prevent or minimize trismus

LLLT/PBM to prevent or reduce the severity of RT-induced trismus in HNC patients has not been reported. The potential of LLLT/PBM to reduce fibrosis and to promote muscle regeneration forms the main rationale for a potential clinical benefit. LLLT/PBM parameters are proposed in table 1.9.

Section 10. Osteoradionecrosis

Soft tissue necrosis and/or osteoradionecrosis (ORN) may occur as a consequence of RT. ORN is a process of radiation-induced vascular occlusion leading to loss of osteocytes and bone necrosis following RT. The incidence of ORN has declined with proper pre-treatment dental care and advances in RT. In conventional RT, mandibular ORN prevalence ranges from 5%–15%, but with the advent of IMRT less than 5% of patients are affected.

The pathogenesis of ORN is not completely understood. It has been proposed that ORN occurs following a radiation-induced fibroatrophic process, including free radical formation, endothelial dysfunction, inflammation, microvascular thrombosis, remodelling, and finally bone and tissue necrosis. Common triggers of necrosis are inflammatory dental disease, trauma to soft tissue, and dental surgical procedures in sites of high dose radiation exposure to bone. Removing of diseased teeth after RT is considered a critical risk factor for ORN, but the lesion can also emerge due to periodontal disease, trauma or even spontaneously. Prevention of ORN is mainly based on extractions of compromised teeth before RT and adequate dental care during and following cancer therapy.

Table 1.9. Trismus treatment parameters. TMJ = temporomandibular joint.

Trismus	*Prophylactic:* *Radiotherapy*: Apply PBM on pterygoid/TMJ region, at least 3 times a week, when high dose RT is given in that region (oropharyngeal and nasopharyngeal carcinoma for example). *Therapeutic*: Continue treatment from the day of diagnosis at least 2 or 3 times a week	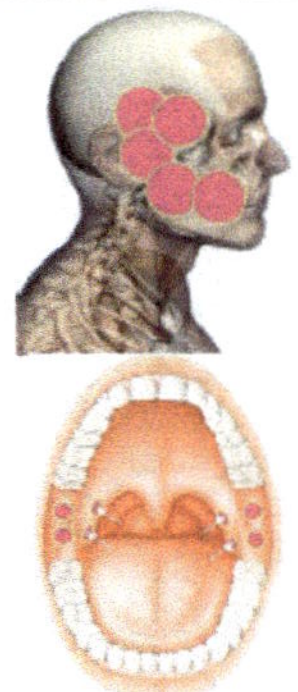	*Extra-oral*: IR laser diodes or LED cluster 750–830 nm 20–80 mW cm^{-2} *Intra-oral*: 630–680 nm 20–200 mW	*Extra-oral*: 3–6 J cm^{-2} laser diodes or LED cluster *Intra-oral*: 3 J per point	*Extra-oral*: Bilaterally over the temporalis muscle, TMJ, masseter muscle. buccinator muscle *Intra-oral*: Bilaterally, point over the region of pterygoids/ pterygomandibular raphae (may be difficultclinically) and other muscles of mastication

Table 1.10. Osteoradionecrosis treatment parameters.

Osteonecrosis	*Therapeutic*: Continue treatment at least 2 or 3 times a week until symptoms improve Daily treatment is recommended Combination with other medical/surgical treatment approaches may be needed.	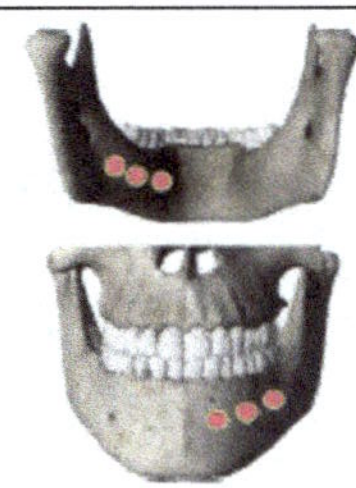	*Extra-oral*: IR laser diodes or LED duster 750–830 nm 20–80 mW cm^{-2} *Intra-oral*: 630–680 nm 20–200 mW	*Extra-oral*: 6 J cm^{-2} laser diodes or LED cluster *Intra-oral*: 6 J per point	*Intra-oral*: Five or more points (1 cm apart) along lingual and buccal aspects of maxilla and/or mandible depending on site and size of region affected

Bevacizumab, an antibody that blocks vascular endothelial growth factor may induce jaw osteonecrosis, possibly as a result of tissue ischemia. Bevacizumab may impair wound healing and can cause osteonecrosis exposed through an oral mucosal. Sunitinib, a TKI that blocks several pathways central to angiogenesis and tumour cell proliferation, has also been associated with osteonecrosis of the jaw.

LLLT/PBM had a biostimulation effect on irradiated rat bone when applied before and during RT. However, an *in vivo* study found that LLLT/PBM was not able to reverse RT-induced bone damage. To our knowledge there are no clinical studies on the effects of LLLT/PBM for RT-induced jaw osteonecrosis. There are several reports on a benefit from LLLT/PBM in the management of bisphosphonate-related osteonecrosis of the jaw (BRONJ) and a proposed prophylactic protocol including LLLT/PBM for reducing BRONJ incidence following tooth extractions. *In vivo* study on rodent wound healing model found evidence that both laser and LED were capable of stimulating angiogenesis. These findings point to a possible role of LLLT/PBM in the management of jaw osteonecrosis induced by RT or angiogenesis inhibitors. We propose LLLT/PBM parameters for future clinical trials in table 1.10.

Section 11. Safety concerns

As with any device used in medicine, safety checks are paramount for LLLT/PBM, in particular if it is to be used as a 'prescribable' therapy for cancer patients. In the past three decades of LLLT/PBM use in the management of OM in cancer patients, no significant adverse effects have been reported. However, the hypothesis that LLLT/PBM has an effect on tumour cells, or protects them from cytotoxic treatment, has been proposed. This section will review what is known to the scientific community so far and what needs to be done to test the above hypotheses.

It is unlikely that LLLT/PBM has carcinogenic effects in normal cells. The non-ionizing wavelengths of the red and NIR spectrum used in LLLT/PBM are far longer than the safety limit of 320 nm for DNA damage. No signs of malignant transformation in non-malignant epithelial cells and fibroblasts were observed following exposure to LLLT/PBM with a wavelength of 660 nm, 350 mW for 15 min during three consecutive days. In addition, no malignant transformation of normal breast epithelial cells was detected in an *in vitro* study comparing the effects of different doses and wavelengths of LLLT/PBM during multiple exposures.

There are no data to suggest that LLLT/PBM may protect cancer cells against the cytotoxic effects of RT or CT. We know that, *in vitro*, LLLT/PBM on RT-induced cytotoxicity in normal and leukemic cells enhances the radiation-induced killing of the malignant cells after LLLT/PBM exposure. Also a pro-apoptotic effect of LLLT/PBM in oral SCC cells has been found, with no anti-apoptotic effects that might promote tumour cell resistance to cancer therapy. Increased apoptosis of human osteosarcoma cells was also induced by the administration of NIR (810 nm, continuous wave, 20 mW cm^{-2}, 1.5 J cm^{-2}) prior to NPe6-mediated photodynamic therapy, as a result of increased cellular ATP and a higher uptake of the photo-sensitiser. LLLT/PBM increased the loco-regional blood flow that contributed to better local oxygenation, and hypothesized that LLLT/PBM applied shortly before cancer treatment might enhance the effect of ionizing RT and local CT.

Most of the effects of LLLT/PBM on cell proliferation and differentiation have been investigated *in vitro* using malignant cell lines, which have generated conflicting data across a range of different tumour cell lines and LLLT/PBM parameters. For example, (i) proliferation of laryngeal carcinoma cells after 809 nm GaAIAs laser irradiation at energy densities between 1.96 and 7.84 J cm^{-2} and (ii) increased cell proliferation of HEp2 carcinoma cells after LLLT/PBM exposure at different wavelengths (685 and 830 nm) and doses. In a study comparing LLLT/PBM administered to normal osteoblasts and to osteosarcoma cells with a range of different wavelengths and doses, only 10 J cm^{-2} from an 830 nm laser was able to enhance osteoblast proliferation, whereas energy densities of 1, 5 and 10 J cm^{-2} from a 780 nm laser decreased proliferation. Osteosarcoma cells were unaffected by 830 nm laser irradiation, whereas a 670 nm laser had a mild proliferative effect. An *in vitro* study compared the effects of different doses of LLLT/PBM at various wavelengths on human breast carcinoma and melanoma cell lines, and found that doses of LLLT/PBM increased breast carcinoma cell proliferation, multiple exposures had either no effect or showed negative dose response relationships. LLLT/PBM (wavelength = 660 nm) administered in low doses (1 J cm^{-2}) increased the *in vitro* proliferation and invasive potential of tongue SCC cells. Similarly, another *in vitro* study suggested that LLLT/PBM (660 or 780 nm, 40 mW, 2.05, 3.07 or 6.15 J cm^{-2}) may stimulate oral dysplastic and oral cancer cells by modulating the Akt/mTOR/CyclinD1 signalling pathway to produce more aggressive behaviour.

In contrast, a decreased mitotic rate was found in gingival SCC after LLLT/PBM at 805 nm and energy density of 4 and 20 J cm^{-2}, whereas no effect on cell proliferation or protein expression of osteosarcoma cells was found when LLLT/PBM was administered with a wavelength of 830 nm. LLLT/PBM (808 nm; 5.85 and 7.8 J cm^{-2}) had an inhibitory effect on the proliferation of a human hepatoma cells line. Glioblastoma/astrocytoma cells exhibited a slightly decreased mitotic rate after LLLT/PBM at 805 nm and 5–20 J cm^{-2}. Similarly, 808 nm laser irradiation with an energy density of more than 5 J cm^{-2} inhibited cell proliferation of glioblastoma cells *in vitro*. Moreover, observed growth inhibition of cancer cell lines occurred at relatively high cumulative LLLT doses. This in fact led to a proposal that, LLLT/PBM may have therapeutic potential in lung cancer. LLLT/PBM administered at a dose of 150 J cm^{-2} appeared to be safe, with only minor effects on B16F10 melanoma cell proliferation *in vitro*, and had no significant effect on tumour growth *in vivo*. Only a high power density (2.5 W cm^{-2}) combined with a very high dose of 1050 J cm^{-2} could induce melanoma tumour growth *in vivo*. LLLT/PBM (660 nm, 30 mW, 424 mW cm^{-2}, 56.4 J cm^{-2}, 133 s, 4 J) applied to chemically induced oral SCC in hamster cheek pouch tissue, increased the growth and severity of the SCC. However, the results were different in a mouse model used to study the effects of LLLT/PBM on multiple UV-induced skin tumours. The experimental mice received full body 670 nm LLLT/PBM delivered twice a day at 5 J cm^{-2} for 37 days, whereas controls received sham LLLT/PBM. No enhanced tumour growth was observed: there was a small but significant reduction in tumour area in the LLLT/PBM group, potentially related to a local photodynamic effect or LLLT/PBM-induced antitumor immune activity. Similar results were reported in an animal study showing that small tumours exposed to LLLT/PBM receded and completely disappeared.

It was hypothesized that upregulation of ATP signalling by LLLT/PBM promoted apoptosis, as well as differentiation of tumour cells, thereby slowing down tumour proliferation.

The results from these studies suggest that different tumour cells have distinct responses to specific LLLT/PBM parameters and doses. In part, these differences may also be explained by variations in the cellular microenvironment, since these have been shown to affect cellular signal transduction pathways to LLLT/PBM exposure. The microenvironment of tumour cells varies among *in vitro* studies and differs significantly from that found in animal models. Moreover, this difference implies that the potential of LLLT/PBM to enhance proliferation of tumour cells *in vitro* does not necessarily translate into harmful effects of LLLT/PBM in cancer patients.

A clinical study reported no differences in cancer recurrence rates for patients receiving LLLT/PBM for lymphedema following breast cancer treatment, compared to controls. A recent RCT in which LLLT/PBM was administered for prevention of OM during CRT in HNC patients (diagnosed with SCC of the nasopharynx, oropharynx and hypopharynx), reported that at a median follow-up of 18 months (range 10–48 months), patients treated with LLLT/PBM had better loco-regional disease control and improved progression-free or overall survival.

Current evidence suggests that LLLT/PBM in the red or NIR spectrum with an energy density of 1–6 J cm^{-2} is safe and effective, hence it should not be withheld, in particular from HNC patients. Nevertheless, as robust evidence for the lack of malignant cell protection or enhancement of tumour growth has not been published, vigilance remains warranted. Further investigations using animal models and long term follow-up (and retrospective analysis) clinical investigations should be conducted to confirm the effects of LLLT/PBM on oncology outcomes and to obtain more insight into dose relationships and the mechanisms of host–tumour responses to LLLT/PBM.

A recent review has identified several biological pathways and molecules involved in the above, in particular for PBM over an area where the tumour has been, resected such as in the case of HNC. While many clinical follow-ups and laboratory studies are warranted in streamlining dose parameters, there are no reported cases of PBM as a source of reactivation of tumour cells in the literature

Section 12. Conclusion and future directions

Acute and chronic complications induced by RT and CRT in patients with HNC represent a significant clinical challenge. There are similarities with respect to pathophysiology across different complications, and patients may suffer from multiple concurrent and interrelated problems. There is anecdotal evidence suggesting that the inflammation associated with acute complications is a harbinger for chronic complications. This observation suggests that preventive approaches starting before, and in the early phases of treatment with RT and CRT, may reduce not only the risk of developing acute problems, but may also have an impact on the risk for late complications.

PBM has shown effectiveness in the management of OM, and elicits several potentially beneficial effects, including reduction of inflammation and pain, promotion of tissue repair, reduction of fibrosis, and protection and regeneration of nerves. Therefore, there is a clear motivation for the application of PBM to treat a broad range of acute and chronic complications associated with RT or CRT in HNC patients and other cancer patients including HSC. RCTs should be conducted to assess the feasibility and efficacy of PBM for prophylactic and therapeutic management of the head and neck complications of cancer therapy.

We hope that this book will serve as the basis for establishing a platform for facilitating future collaborations among clinicians and researchers, which will then create firm scientific evidence for the use of PBM in patients with HNC. PBM protocols should be administered using suitable parameters for the anatomic structures at risk. The parameters (including the wavelengths) we have proposed are largely based on evidence derived from studies using PBM for the management of OM (typically 633–685 nm or 780–830 nm). However, trials directed to other (non-head and neck) indications for the use of PBM suggest that a broader range of wavelengths (590–1064 nm) has efficacy for healing and for reducing inflammation and pain. Future investigations should be conducted to better define optimal PBM parameters for each of the complications of HNC treatment. In addition, the ideal timing and frequency of PBM administration should be determined, as well as how long PBM should be continued following the completion of cancer treatment. PBM parameters should be reported in detail (as discussed in section 1). Validated outcome measures must be identified and employed to assess the effect of prophylaxis and therapy, from the time of diagnosis through active treatment and survival.

With regard to HNC, bearing in mind the reasonable safety and potential benefits, one must be cautious when considering the possibility of residual tumours within the site of PBM. While the reported results of *in vitro* studies of PBM on malignant cells vary, and clinical reports have shown little or no adverse reactions, there is a paucity of robust data regarding potential protection and promotion of tumours. Studies should also be directed toward the potential beneficial effects of PBM by enhancing the efficacy of (C)RT or immunologic antitumor reactivity. It is thus imperative that further investigations be aimed at obtaining more insight into the mechanisms of the host–tumour responses to PBM and to elucidating the effects of PBM on oncology treatment outcomes.

Bibliography

Al-Dasooqi N *et al* 2013 Emerging evidence on the pathobiology of mucositis *Support. Care Cancer* **21** 3233–41

Al-Watban F A and Andres B L 2012 Laser biomodulation of normal and neoplastic cells *Lasers Med. Sci.* **27** 1039–43

Antunes F, Boveris A and Cadenas E 2004 On the mechanism and biology of cytochrome oxidase inhibition by nitric oxide *Proc. Natl Acad. Sci. USA* **101** 16774–9

Antunes H S *et al* 2013 Phase III trial of low-level laser therapy to prevent oral mucositis in head and neck cancer patients treated with concurrent chemoradiation *Radiother. Oncol.* **109** 297–302

Aras M H and Gungormus M 2010 Placebo-controlled randomized clinical trial of the effect two different low-level laser therapies (LLLT)—intraoral and extraoral—on trismus and facial swelling following surgical extraction of the lower third molar *Lasers Med. Sci.* **25** 641–5

Arbabi-Kalati F, Arbabi-Kalati F and Moridi T 2013 Evaluation of the effect of low level laser on prevention of chemotherapy-induced mucositis *Acta Med. Iran.* **51** 157–62

Assis L, Moretti A I, Abrahao T B, Cury V, Souza H P, Hamblin M R and Parizotto N A 2012 Low-level laser therapy (808 nm) reduces inflammatory response and oxidative stress in rat tibialis anterior muscle after cryolesion *Lasers Surg. Med.* **44** 726–35

Avci P *et al* 2013 Low-level laser (light) therapy (LLLT) in skin: stimulating, healing, restoring *Semin. Cutan. Med. Surg.* **32** 41–52

Avila J L, Grundmann O, Burd R and Limesand K H 2009 Radiation-induced salivary gland dysfunction results from p53-dependent apoptosis *Int. J. Radiat. Oncol. Biol. Phys.* **73** 523–9

Bagan J V *et al* 2009 Osteonecrosis of the jaws by intravenous bisphosphonates and osteoradionecrosis: a comparative study *Med. Oral Patol. Oral Cir. Bucal.* **14** e616–e9

Barasch A, Raber-Durlacher J, Epstein J B and Carroll J 2015 Effects of pre-radiation exposure to LLLT of normal and malignant cells *Support. Care Cancer* **24** 2497–501

Barolet D and Boucher A 2010 Prophylactic low-level light therapy for the treatment of hypertrophic scars and keloids: a case series *Lasers Surg. Med.* **42** 597–601

Batista J D, Zanetta-Barbosa D, Cardoso S V, Dechichi P, Rocha F S and Pagnoncelli R M 2014 Effect of low-level laser therapy on repair of the bone compromised by radiotherapy *Lasers Med. Sci.* **29** 1913–8

Bensadoun R J and Nair R G 2012 Low-level laser therapy in the prevention and treatment of cancer therapy-induced mucositis: 2012 state of the art based on literature review and meta-analysis *Curr. Opin. Oncol.* **24** 363–70

Bensadoun R J and Nair R G 2015 Low-level laser therapy in the management of mucositis and dermatitis induced by cancer therapy *Photomed. Laser Surg.* **33** 487–91

Bensadoun R J, Riesenbeck D, Lockhart P B, Elting L S, Spijkervet F K and Brennan M T 2010 A systematic review of trismus induced by cancer therapies in head and neck cancer patients *Support. Care Cancer.* **18** 1033–8

Bernier J *et al* 2008 Consensus guidelines for the management of radiation dermatitis and coexisting acne-like rash in patients receiving radiotherapy plus EGFR inhibitors for the treatment of squamous cell carcinoma of the head and neck *Ann. Oncol.* **19** 142–9

Bjordal J M 2012 Low level laser therapy (LLLT) and world association for laser therapy (WALT) dosage recommendations *Photomed. Laser Surg.* **30** 61–2

Bjordal J M, Bensadoun R J, Tuner J, Frigo L, Gjerde K and Lopes-Martins R A 2011 A systematic review with meta-analysis of the effect of low-level laser therapy (LLLT) in cancer therapy-induced oral mucositis *Support. Care Cancer* **19** 1069–77

Bjordal J M, Couppe C, Chow R T, Tuner J and Ljunggren E A 2003 A systematic review of low level laser therapy with location-specific doses for pain from chronic joint disorders *Aust. J. Physiother.* **49** 107–16

Bjordal J M, Johnson M I, Iversen V, Aimbire F and Lopes-Martins R A 2006 Low-level laser therapy in acute pain: a systematic review of possible mechanisms of action and clinical effects in randomized placebo-controlled trials *Photomed. Laser Surg.* **24** 158–168

Boltong A *et al* 2014 A prospective cohort study of the effects of adjuvant breast cancer chemotherapy on taste function, food liking, appetite and associated nutritional outcomes *PLoS One* **9** e103512

Buglione M *et al* 2016 Oral toxicity management in head and neck cancer patients treated with chemotherapy and radiation: dental pathologies and osteoradionecrosis (Part 1) literature review and consensus statement *Crit. Rev. Oncol./Hematol.* **97** 131–42

Burlage F R, Coppes R P, Meertens H, Stokman M A and Vissink A 2001 Parotid and submandibular/sublingual salivary flow during high dose radiotherapy *Radiother. Oncol.* **61** 271–4

Carnaby-Mann G, Crary M A, Schmalfuss I and Amdur R 2012 "Pharyngocise": randomized controlled trial of preventative exercises to maintain muscle structure and swallowing function during head-and-neck chemoradiotherapy *Int. J. Radiat. Oncol. Biol. Phys.* **83** 210–9

Carrillo J S, Calatayud J, Manso F J, Barberia E, Martinez J M and Donado M 1990 A randomized double-blind clinical trial on the effectiveness of helium–neon laser in the prevention of pain, swelling and trismus after removal of impacted third molars *Int. Dent. J.* **40** 31–6

Chang L, Graham P H, Hao J, Ni J, Bucci J, Cozzi P J, Kearsley J H and Li Y 2013 Acquisition of epithelial-mesenchymal transition and cancer stem cell phenotypes is associated with activation of the PI3K/Akt/mTOR pathway in prostate cancer radioresistance *Cell Death Dis.* **4** e875

Chen Y K, Huang A H, Cheng P H, Yang S H and Lin L M 2013 Overexpression of Smad proteins, especially Smad7, in oral epithelial dysplasias *Clin. Oral Investig.* **17** 921–32

Chow R T, Johnson M I, Lopes-Martins R A and Bjordal J M 2009 Efficacy of low-level laser therapy in the management of neck pain: a systematic review and meta-analysis of randomised placebo or active-treatment controlled trials *Lancet* **374** 1897–908

Chow R, Armati P, Laakso E L, Bjordal J M and Baxter G D 2011 Inhibitory effects of laser irradiation on peripheral mammalian nerves and relevance to analgesic effects: a systematic review *Photomed. Laser Surg.* **29** 365–81

Chrcanovic B R, Reher P, Sousa A A and Harris M 2010 Osteoradionecrosis of the jaws—a current overview—part 1: physiopathology and risk and predisposing factors *Oral Maxillofac. Surg.* **14** 3–16

Chung H, Dai T, Sharma S K, Huang Y Y, Carroll J D and Hamblin M R 2012 The nuts and bolts of low-level laser (light) therapy *Ann. Biomed. Eng.* **40** 516–33

Clarkson J E, Worthington H V, Furness S, McCabe M, Khalid T and Meyer S 2010 Interventions for treating oral mucositis for patients with cancer receiving treatment *Cochrane Database Syst. Rev.* **2010** CD001973

Coombe A R, Ho C T, Darendeliler M A, Hunter N, Philips J R, Chapple C C and Yum L W 2001 The effects of low level laser irradiation on osteoblastic cells *Clin. Orthod. Res.* **4** 3–14

Cooperstein E *et al* 2012 Vanderbilt head and neck symptom survey version 2.0: report of the development and initial testing of a subscale for assessment of oral health *Head Neck* **34** 797–804

Costa M M, Silva S B, Quinto A L, Pasquinelli P F, de Queiroz dos Santos V, de Cássia Santos G and Veiga D F 2014 Phototherapy 660 nm for the prevention of radiodermatitis in breast cancer patients receiving radiation therapy: study protocol for a randomized controlled trial *Trials* **15** 330

Cowen D, Tardieu C, Schubert M, Peterson D, Resbeut M, Faucher C and Franquin J C 1997 Low energy helium–neon laser in the prevention of oral mucositis in patients undergoing bone marrow transplant: results of a double blind randomized trial *Int. J. Radiat. Oncol. Biol. Phys.* **38** 697–703

Crous A M and Abrahamse H 2013 Lung cancer stem cells and low-intensity laser irradiation: a potential future therapy? *Stem Cell Res. Ther.* **4** 129

Cui X *et al* 2014 Significance of elevated ERK expression and its positive correlation with EGFR in kazakh patients with esophageal squamous cell carcinoma *Int. J. Clin. Exp. Pathol.* **7** 2382–91 PMCID: PMC4069965

Da Cunha S S *et al* 2007 Effect of laser therapy on bone tissue submitted to radiotherapy: experimental study in rats *Photomed. Laser Surg.* **25** 197–204

da Guarda M G, Paraguassu G M, Cerqueira N S, Cury P R, Farias J G and Ramalho L M 2012 Laser GaAlAs (λ860 nm) photobiomodulation for the treatment of bisphosphonate-induced osteonecrosis of the jaw *Photomed. Laser Surg.* **30** 293–7

Dang Y, Liu B, Liu L, Ye X, Bi X, Zhang Y and Gu J 2011 The 800-nm diode laser irradiation induces skin collagen synthesis by stimulating TGF-β/Smad signaling pathway *Lasers Med. Sci.* **26** 837–43

de Castro J L, Pinheiro A L, Werneck C E and Soares C P 2005 The effect of laser therapy on the proliferation of oral KB carcinoma cells: an *in vitro* study *Photomed. Laser Surg.* **23** 586–9

de Lima F M, Villaverde A B, Albertini R, Correa J C, Carvalho R L, Munin E, Araujo T, Silva J A and Aimbire F 2011 Dual Effect of low-level laser therapy (LLLT) on the acute lung inflammation induced by intestinal ischemia and reperfusion: action on anti- and pro-inflammatory cytokines *Lasers Surg. Med.* **43** 410–20

de Sousa A P *et al* 2013 Laser and LED phototherapies on angiogenesis *Lasers Med. Sci* **28** 981–7

de C, Monteiro J S, Pinheiro A N, de Oliveira S C, Aciole G T, Sousa J A, Canguss M C and Dos Santos J N 2011 Influence of laser phototherapy (λ660 nm) on the outcome of oral chemical carcinogenesis on the hamster cheek pouch model: histological study *Photomed. Laser Surg.* **29** 741–5

DeLand M M, Weiss R A, McDaniel D H and Geronemus R G 2007 Treatment of radiation-induced dermatitis with light-emitting diode (LED) photomodulation *Lasers Surg. Med.* **39** 164–8

Delanian S and Lefaix J L 2004 The radiation-induced fibroatrophic process: therapeutic perspective via the antioxidant pathway *Radiother. Oncol.* **73** 119–31

Deng J *et al* 2012a Factors associated with external and internal lymphedema in patients with head-and-neck cancer *Int. J. Radiat. Oncol. Biol. Phys.* **84** e319–e28

Deng J *et al* 2012b Prevalence of secondary lymphedema in patients with head and neck cancer *J. Pain Symptom. Manage.* **43** 244–52

Deng J, Ridner S H, Aulino J M and Murphy B A 2015 Assessment and measurement of head and neck lymphedema: state-of-the-science and future directions *Oral Oncol.* **51** 431–7

Deng J, Ridner S H and Murphy B A 2011 Lymphedema in patients with head and neck cancer *Oncol. Nurs. Forum.* **38** E1–E10

Dhillon A S, Hagan S, Rath O and Kolch W 2007 MAP kinase signalling pathways in cancer *Oncogene* **26** 3279–90

Dijkstra P U, Huisman P M and Roodenburg J L 2006 Criteria for trismus in head and neck oncology *Int. J. Oral Maxillofac. Surg.* **35** 337–42

Dijkstra P U, Kalk W W and Roodenburg J L 2004 Trismus in head and neck oncology: a systematic review *Oral Oncol.* **40** 879–89

Dirican A, Andacoglu O, Johnson R, McGuire K, Mager L and Soran A 2011 The short-term effects of low-level laser therapy in the management of breast-cancer-related lymphedema *Support. Care Cancer* **19** 685–90

Dorr W and Hendry J H 2001 Consequential late effects in normal tissues *Radiother. Oncol.* **61** 223–31

Dwivedi R C *et al* 2009 Evaluation of speech outcomes following treatment of oral and oropharyngeal cancers *Cancer Treat. Rev.* **35** 417–24

Eisbruch A *et al* 2002 Objective assessment of swallowing dysfunction and aspiration after radiation concurrent with chemotherapy for head-and-neck cancer *Int. J. Radiat. Oncol. Biol. Phys.* **53** 23–8

El-Maghraby E M, El-Rouby D H and Saafan A M 2013 Assessment of the effect of low-energy diode laser irradiation on gamma irradiated rats' mandibles *Arch. Oral Biol.* **58** 796–805

Elting L S *et al* 2008 Patient-reported measurements of oral mucositis in head and neck cancer patients treated with radiotherapy with or without chemotherapy: demonstration of increased frequency, severity, resistance to palliation, and impact on quality of life *Cancer* **113** 2704–13

Epstein J B *et al* 2012 Oral complications of cancer and cancer therapy: from cancer treatment to survivorship *CA Cancer J. Clin.* **62** 400–22

Epstein J B and Barasch A 2010 Taste disorders in cancer patients: pathogenesis, and approach to assessment and management *Oral Oncol.* **46** 77–81

Epstein J B, Robertson M, Emerton S, Phillips N and Stevenson-Moore P 2001 Quality of life and oral function in patients treated with radiation therapy for head and neck cancer *Head Neck* **23** 389–98

Epstein J B, Thariat J, Bensadoun R J, Barasch A, Murphy B A, Kolnick L, Popplewell L and Maghami E 2012 Oral complications of cancer and cancer therapy: from cancer treatment to survivorship *CA Cancer J. Clin.* **62** 400–22

Epstein J, van der Meij E, McKenzie M, Wong F, Lepawsky M and Stevenson-Moore P 1997 Postradiation osteonecrosis of the mandible: a long-term follow-up study *Oral Surg Oral Med. Oral Pathol. Oral Radiol. Endodontics* **83** 657–62

Feng J, Zhang Y and Xing D 2012 Low-power laser irradiation (LPLI) promotes VEGF expression and vascular endothelial cell proliferation through the activation of ERK/Sp1 pathway *Cell Signal* **24** 1116–25

Fife D *et al* 2010 A randomized, controlled, double-blind study of light emitting diode photo-modulation for the prevention of radiation dermatitis in patients with breast cancer. *Dermatol. Surg.* **36** 1921–7

Fillipin L I, Mauriz J L, Vedovelli K, Moreira A J, Zettler C G, Lech O, Marroni N P and Gonzalez-Gallego J 2005 Low-level laser therapy (LLLT) prevents oxidative stress and reduces fibrosis in rat traumatized achilles tendon *Lasers Surg. Med.* **37** 293–300

Frigo L, Luppi J S, Favero G M, Maria D A, Penna S C, Bjordal J M, Bensadoun R J and Lopes-Martins RA 2009 The effect of low-level laser irradiation (In–Ga–Al–AsP 660 nm) on melanoma *in vitro* and *in vivo BMC Cancer* **9** 404

Fujimaki Y, Shimoyama T, Liu Q, Umeda T, Nakaji S and Sugawara K 2003 Low-level laser irradiation attenuates production of reactive oxygen species by human neutrophils *J. Clin. Laser Med. Surg.* **21** 165–70

Ganzer H, Touger-Decker R, Parrott J S, Murphy B A, Epstein J B and Huhmann M B 2013 Symptom burden in head and neck cancer: impact upon oral energy and protein intake *Support. Care Cancer* **21** 495–503

Gautam A P, Fernandes D J, Vidyasagar M S, Maiya A G and Vadhiraja B M 2012 Low level laser therapy for concurrent chemoradiotherapy induced oral mucositis in head and neck cancer patients—a triple blinded randomized controlled trial *Radiother. Oncol.* **104** 349–54

Gobbo M, Ottaviani G, Mustacchi G, Di Lenarda R and Biasotto M 2012 Acneiform rash due to epidermal growth factor receptor inhibitors: high-level laser therapy as an innovative approach *Lasers Med. Sci.* **27** 1085–90

Goldstein M, Maxymiw W G, Cummings B J and Wood R E 1999 The effects of antitumor irradiation on mandibular opening and mobility: a prospective study of 58 patients *Oral Surg. Oral Med. Oral Pathol. Oral Radiol. Endodontics* **88** 365–73

Gomes Henriques Á C, Ginani F, Oliveira R M, Keesen T S, Galvão Barboza C A, Oliveira Rocha H A, de Castro J F, Della Coletta R and de Almeida Freitas R 2014 Low-level laser therapy promotes proliferation and invasion of oral squamous cell carcinoma cells *Lasers Med Sci.* **29** 1385–95

Guirro R R and Weis L C 2009 Radiant power determination of low-level laser therapy equipment and characterization of its clinical use procedures *Photomed. Laser Surg.* **27** 633–9

Gupta A, Keshri G K, Yadav A, Gola S, Chauhan S, Salhan A K and Bala Singh S 2014 Superpulsed (Ga-As, 904 nm) low-level laser therapy (LLLT) attenuates inflammatory response and enhances healing of burn wounds *J. Biophotonics* **8** 489

Hashmi J T, Huang Y Y, Sharma S K, Kurup D B, De T L, Carroll J D and Hamblin M R 2010 Effect of pulsing in low-level light therapy *Lasers Surg. Med.* **42** 450–66

Hawkins D and Abrahamse H 2005 Biological effects of helium–neon laser irradiation on normal and wounded human skin fibroblasts *Photomed. Laser Surg.* **23** 251–9

Hodgson B D, Margolis D M, Salzman D E, Eastwood D, Tarima S, Williams L D, Sande J E, Vaughan W P and Whelan H T 2012 Amelioration of oral mucositis pain by NASA near-infrared light-emitting diodes in bone marrow transplant patients *Support. Care Cancer* **20** 1405–15

Hovan A J *et al* 2010 A systematic review of dysgeusia induced by cancer therapies *Support. Care Cancer* **18** 1081–7

Huang Y Y, Chen A C, Carroll J D and Hamblin M R 2009 Biphasic dose response in low level light therapy *Dose Response* **7** 358–83

Huang Y Y, Sharma S K, Carroll J and Hamblin M R 2011 Biphasic dose response in low level light therapy—an update *Dose Response* **9** 602–18

Hudson D E, Hudson D O, Wininger J M and Richardson B D 2013 Penetration of laser light at 808 and 980 nm in bovine tissue samples *Photomed. Laser Surg.* **31** 163–8

Hunter K U *et al* 2013 Toxicities affecting quality of life after chemo-IMRT of oropharyngeal cancer: prospective study of patient-reported, observer-rated, and objective outcomes *Int. J. Radiat. Oncol. Biol. Phys.* **85** 935–40

Hwang Y S, Park K K and Chung W Y 2014 Stromal transforming growth factor-β1 is crucial for reinforcing the invasive potential of low invasive cancer *Arch. Oral Biol.* **59** 687–94

Hymes S R, Strom E A and Fife C 2006 Radiation dermatitis: clinical presentation, pathophysiology, and treatment 2006 *J. Am. Acad. Dermatol.* **54** 28–46

Jacobi I, Navran A, van der Molen L, Heemsbergen W D, Hilgers F J and van den Brekel M W 2015 Radiation dose to the tongue and velopharynx predicts acoustic-articulatory changes after chemo-IMRT treatment for advanced head and neck cancer *Eur. Arch. Otorhinolaryngol.* **273** 487–94

Jacobi I, van der Molen L, Huiskens H, van Rossum M A and Hilgers F J 2010 Voice and speech outcomes of chemoradiation for advanced head and neck cancer: a systematic review *Eur. Arch. Otorhinolaryngol.* **267** 1495–505

Jenkins P A and Carroll J D 2011 How to report low-level laser therapy (LLLT)/photomedicine dose and beam parameters in clinical and laboratory studies *Photomed. Laser Surg.* **29** 785–7

Jensen S B *et al* 2010 A systematic review of salivary gland hypofunction and xerostomia induced by cancer therapies: prevalence, severity and impact on quality of life *Support. Care Cancer* **18** 1039–60

Johns M M, Kolachala V, Berg E, Muller S, Creighton F X and Branski R C 2012 Radiation fibrosis of the vocal fold: from man to mouse *Laryngoscope* **122**(Suppl 5) S107–S25

Karu T I 2010 Multiple roles of cytochrome c oxidase in mammalian cells under action of red and IR-A radiation *IUBMB Life* **62** 607–10

Karu T I and Kolyakov S F 2005 Exact action spectra for cellular responses relevant to phototherapy *Photomed. Laser Surg.* **23** 355–61

Karu T I, Pyatibrat L V and Kalendo G S 2004 Photobiological modulation of cell attachment via cytochrome c oxidase *Photochem. Photobiol. Sci.* **3** 211–6

Karu T 1989 Photobiology of low-power laser effects *Health Phys.* **56** 691–704

Kawano Y, Utsunomiya-Kai Y, Kai K, Miyakawa I, Ohshiro T and Narahara H 2012 The production of VEGF involving MAP kinase activation by low level laser therapy in human granulosa cells *Laser Ther.* **21** 269–74

Khakh B S and Burnstock G 2009 The double life of ATP *Sci. Am.* **301**(84–90) 92

Kim J H, Kolozsvary A J, Jenrow K A and Brown S L 2013 Mechanisms of radiation-induced skin injury and implications for future clinical trials *Int. J. Radiat. Biol.* **89** 311–8

Kraaijenga S A, Oskam I M, van der Molen L, Hamming-Vrieze O, Hilgers F J and van den Brekel MW 2015 Evaluation of long term (10-years+) dysphagia and trismus in patients treated with concurrent chemo-radiotherapy for advanced head and neck cancer *Oral Oncol.* **51** 787–94

Kraaijenga S A, van der Molen L, van den Brekel MW and Hilgers F J 2014 Current assessment and treatment strategies of dysphagia in head and neck cancer patients: a systematic review of the 2012/13 literature *Curr. Opin. Support. Palliative Care* **8** 152–63

Kreisler M, Christoffers A B, Willershausen B and d'Hoedt B 2003 Low-level 809 nm GaAlAs laser irradiation increases the proliferation rate of human laryngeal carcinoma cells *in vitro Lasers Med. Sci.* **18** 100–3

Kushibiki T, Hirasawa T, Okawa S and Ishihara M 2013 Regulation of miRNA expression by low-level laser therapy (LLLT) and photodynamic therapy (PDT) *Int. J. Mol. Sci.* **14** 13542–58

Lacouture M E, Anadkat M J, Bensadoun R J, Bryce J, Chan A, Epstein J B, Eaby-Sandy B and Murphy BA 2011 Clinical practice guidelines for the prevention and treatment of EGFR inhibitor-associated dermatologic toxicities *Support. Care Cancer* **19** 1079–95

Lalla R V *et al* 2014 MASCC/ISOO clinical practice guidelines for the management of mucositis secondary to cancer therapy *Cancer* **120** 1453–61

Langendijk J A, Doornaert P, Rietveld D H, Verdonck-de Leeuw I M, Leemans C R and Slotman B J 2009 A predictive model for swallowing dysfunction after curative radiotherapy in head and neck cancer *Radiother. Oncol.* **90** 189–95

Langendijk J A, Doornaert P, Verdonck-de Leeuw I M, Leemans C R, Aaronson N K and Slotman B J 2008 Impact of late treatment-related toxicity on quality of life among patients with head and neck cancer treated with radiotherapy *J. Clin. Oncol.* **26** 3770–6

Langmore S E 2003 Evaluation of oropharyngeal dysphagia: which diagnostic tool is superior? *Curr. Opin. Otolaryngol. Head Neck Surg.* **11** 485–9

Lau R W and Cheing G L 2009 Managing postmastectomy lymphedema with low-level laser therapy *Photomed. Laser Surg.* **27** 763–9

Leslie P, Carding P N and Wilson J A 2003 Investigation and management of chronic dysphagia *Br. Med. J.* **326** 433–6

Lev-Tov H, Brody N, Siegel D and Jagdeo J 2013 Inhibition of fibroblast proliferation *in vitro* using low-level infrared light-emitting diodes *Dermatol. Surg.* **39** 422–5

Lima MTE, Lima JGE, de Andrade M F and Bergmann A 2012 Low-level laser therapy in secondary lymphedema after breast cancer: systematic review *Lasers Med. Sci.* **29** 1289–95

Liu T C, Zhang J and Li X E 2013 The balance between normal and tumor tissues in phototherapy of tissues harboring cancer *Photomed. Laser Surg.* **31** 93–4

Liu Y H, Cheng C C, Ho C C, Pei R J, Lee K Y, Yeh K T, Chan Y and Lai Y S 2004 Effects of diode 808 nm GaAlAs low-power laser irradiation on inhibition of the proliferation of human hepatoma cells *in vitro* and their possible mechanism *Res. Commun. Mol. Pathol. Pharmacol.* **115–116** 185–201 PMID: 17564317

Lohr N L, Keszler A, Pratt P, Bienengraber M, Warltier D C and Hogg N 2009 Enhancement of nitric oxide release from nitrosyl hemoglobin and nitrosyl myoglobin by red/near infrared radiation: potential role in cardioprotection *J. Mol. Cell Cardiol.* **47** 256–63

Loncar B, Stipetic M M, Baricevic M and Risovic D 2011 The effect of low-level laser therapy on salivary glands in patients with xerostomia *Photomed. Laser Surg.* **29** 171–5

Lopes N N, Plapler H, Chavantes M C, Lalla R V, Yoshimura E M and Alves M T 2009 Cyclooxygenase-2 and vascular endothelial growth factor expression in 5-fluorouracil-induced oral mucositis in hamsters: evaluation of two low-intensity laser protocols *Support. Care Cancer* **17** 1409–15

Lopes N N, Plapler H, Lalla R V, Chavantes M C, Yoshimura E M, da Silva M A and Alves M T 2010 Effects of low-level laser therapy on collagen expression and neutrophil infiltrate in 5-fluorouracil-induced oral mucositis in hamsters *Lasers Surg. Med.* **42** 546–52

Luo L, Sun Z, Zhang L, Li X, Dong Y and Liu TC 2013 Effects of low-level laser therapy on ROS homeostasis and expression of IGF-1 and TGF-β1 in skeletal muscle during the repair process *Lasers Med. Sci.* **28** 725–34

Luomanen M and Alaluusua S 2012 Treatment of bisphosphonate-induced osteonecrosis of the jaws with Nd:YAG laser biostimulation *Lasers Med. Sci.* **27** 251–5

Madrid C, Abarca M and Bouferrache K 2010 Osteoradionecrosis: an update *Oral Oncol.* **46** 471–4

Mancini M L and Sonis S T 2014 Mechanisms of cellular fibrosis associated with cancer regimen-related toxicities *Front. Pharmacol.* **5** 51

Marchesini R, Dasdia T, Melloni E and Rocca E 1989 Effect of low-energy laser irradiation on colony formation capability in different human tumor cells *in vitro Lasers Surg. Med.* **9** 59–62

Marinho R R *et al* 2014 Potential anti-inflammatory effect of low-level laser therapy on the experimental reflux laryngitis: a preliminary study *Lasers Med. Sci.* **29** 239–43

Martin M, Lefaix J and Delanian S 2000 TGF-β1 and radiation fibrosis: a master switch and a specific therapeutic target? *Int. J. Radiat. Oncol. Biol. Phys.* **47** 277–90

McGarvey A C, Osmotherly P G, Hoffman G R and Chiarelli P E 2014 Lymphoedema following treatment for head and neck cancer: impact on patients, and beliefs of health professionals *Eur. J. Cancer Care* **23** 317–27

Meleca R J, Dworkin J P, Kewson D T, Stachler R J and Hill S L 2003 Functional outcomes following nonsurgical treatment for advanced-stage laryngeal carcinoma *Laryngoscope* **113** 720–8

Mendenhall W M, Parsons J T, Buatti J M, Stringer S P, Million R R and Cassisi N J 1995 Advances in radiotherapy for head and neck cancer *Semin. Surg. Oncol.* **11** 256–64

Meneguzzo D T, Lopes L A, Pallota R, Soares-Ferreira L, Lopes-Martins R A and Ribeiro M S 2013 Prevention and treatment of mice paw edema by near-infrared low-level laser therapy on lymph nodes *Lasers Med. Sci.* **28** 973–80

Mester E, Spiry T, Szende B and Tota J G 1971 Effect of laser rays on wound healing *Am. J. Surg.* **122** 532–5

Mester E, Szende B and Gartner P 1968 The effect of laser beams on the growth of hair in mice *Radiobiol. Radiother.* **9** 621–6

Migliorati C, Hewson I, Lalla R V, Antunes H S, Estilo C L, Hodgson B, Lopes N N, Schubert M M, Bowen J and Elad S 2013 Systematic review of laser and other light therapy for the management of oral mucositis in cancer patients *Support. Care Cancer* **21** 333–41

Mittal B B *et al* 2003 Swallowing dysfunction—preventative and rehabilitation strategies in patients with head-and-neck cancers treated with surgery, radiotherapy, and chemotherapy: a critical review *Int. J. Radiat. Oncol. Biol. Phys.* **57** 1219–30

Murayama H, Sadakane K, Yamanoha B and Kogure S 2012 Low-power 808 nm laser irradiation inhibits cell proliferation of a human-derived glioblastoma cell line *in vitro* *Lasers Med. Sci.* **27** 87–93

Murphy B A *et al* 2010 Reliability and validity of the vanderbilt head and neck symptom survey: a tool to assess symptom burden in patients treated with chemoradiation *Head Neck* **32** 26–37

Murphy B A and Gilbert J 2009 Dysphagia in head and neck cancer patients treated with radiation: assessment, sequelae, and rehabilitation *Semin. Radiat. Oncol.* **19** 35–42

Murrell G A, Francis M J and Bromley L 1990 Modulation of fibroblast proliferation by oxygen free radicals *Biochem. J.* **265** 659–65

Myakishev-Rempel M, Stadler I, Brondon P, Axe D R, Friedman M, Nardia F B and Lanzafame R 2012 A preliminary study of the safety of red light phototherapy of tissues harboring cancer *Photomed. Laser Surg.* **30** 551–8

Nagata Y, Takahashi A, Ohnishi K, Ota I, Ohnishi T, Tojo T and Taniguchi S 2010 Effect of rapamycin, an mTOR inhibitor, on radiation sensitivity of lung cancer cells having different p53 gene status *Int. J. Oncol.* **37** 1001–10

Nguyen N P *et al* Aspiration rate following chemoradiation for head and neck cancer: an underreported occurrence *Radiother. Oncol.* **80** 302–6

Nguyen N P *et al* 2007 Effectiveness of the cough reflex in patients with aspiration following radiation for head and neck cancer *Lung* **185** 243–8

Oberoi S, Zamperlini-Netto G, Beyene J, Treister N S and Sung L 2014 Effect of prophylactic low level laser therapy on oral mucositis: a systematic review and meta-analysis *PLoS One* **9** e107418

Ohrn K E, Wahlin Y B and Sjoden P O 2001 Oral status during radiotherapy and chemotherapy: a descriptive study of patient experiences and the occurrence of oral complications *Support. Care Cancer* **9** 247–57

Oliveira F A *et al* 2012 Low-level laser therapy decreases renal interstitial fibrosis *Photomed. Laser Surg.* **30** 705–13

Omar M T, Shaheen A A and Zafar H 2012 A systematic review of the effect of low-level laser therapy in the management of breast cancer-related lymphedema *Support. Care Cancer.* **20** 2977–84

Oron U *et al* 2001 Low-energy laser irradiation reduces formation of scar tissue after myocardial infarction in rats and dogs *Circulation* **103** 296–301

Oton-Leite A F *et al* 2013 Effect of low level laser therapy in the reduction of oral complications in patients with cancer of the head and neck submitted to radiotherapy *Special Care Dentistry* **33** 294–300

Pardali K and Moustakas A 2007 Actions of TGF-β as tumor suppressor and pro-metastatic factor in human cancer *Biochim. Biophys. Acta* **1775** 21–62

Pedersen A M, Bardow A, Jensen S B and Nauntofte B 2002 Saliva and gastrointestinal functions of taste, mastication, swallowing and digestion *Oral Dis.* **8** 117–29

Pellicioli A C, Martins M D, Dillenburg C S, Marques M M, Squarize C H and Castilho R M 2014 Laser phototherapy accelerates oral keratinocyte migration through the modulation of the mammalian target of rapamycin signaling pathway *J. Biomed. Opt.* **19** 028002

Pinheiro A L, Carneiro N S, Vieira A L, Brugnera A Jr, Zanin F A, Barros R A and Silva P S 2002 Effects of low-level laser therapy on malignant cells: *in vitro* study *J. Clin. Laser Med. Surg.* **20** 23–26

Plavnik L M, De Crosa M E and Malberti A I 2003 Effect of low-power radiation (helium/neon) upon submandibulary glands *J. Clin. Laser Med. Surg.* **21** 219–25

Plavnik L M, De Crosa M E and Malberti A I 2003 Irradiation effect of low-energy laser on rat submandibular salivary gland *J. Oral Pathol.* **17** 91–94

Png K J, Halberg N, Yoshida M and Tavazoie S F 2012 A microRNA regulon that mediates endothelial recruitment and metastasis by cancer cells *Nature* **481** 190–4

Powell K, Low P, McDonnell P A, Laakso E L and Ralph S J 2010 The effect of laser irradiation on proliferation of human breast carcinoma, melanoma, and immortalized mammary epithelial cells *Photomed. Laser Surg.* **28** 115–23

Prime S S, Davies M, Pring M and Paterson I C 2004 The role of TGF-β in epithelial malignancy and its relevance to the pathogenesis of oral cancer part II *Crit. Rev. Oral Biol. Med.* **15** 337–47

Raber-Durlacher J E *et al* 2012 Swallowing dysfunction in cancer patients *Support. Care Cancer* **20** 433–43

Raber-Durlacher J E and Scully C 2010 Oral cancer: comprehending the condition, causes, controversies, control and consequences. 14: Mucositis *Dent. Update* **39** 145–7

Rapidis A D, Vermorken J B and Bourhis J 2008 Targeted therapies in head and neck cancer: past, present and future. *Rev. Recent Clin. Trials* **3** 156–66

Renno A C, McDonnell P A, Parizotto N A and Laakso E L 2007 The effects of laser irradiation on osteoblast and osteosarcoma cell proliferation and differentiation *in vitro Photomed. Laser Surg.* **25** 275–280

Rezvani M, Robbins M E, Hopewell J W and Whitehouse E M 1993 Modification of late dermal necrosis in the pig by treatment with multi-wavelength light *Br. J. Radiol.* **66** 145–9

Rizzi C F, Mauriz J L, Freitas Correa D S, Moreira A J, Zettler C G, Filippin L I, Marroni N P and Gonzalez-Gallego J 2006 Effects of low-level laser therapy (LLLT) on the nuclear factor (NF)-κB signaling pathway in traumatized muscle *Lasers Surg. Med.* **38** 704–13

Roe J W *et al* 2010 Swallowing outcomes following Intensity Modulated Radiation Therapy (IMRT) for head and neck cancer—a systematic review *Oral Oncol.* **46** 727–33

Romeo U *et al* 2011 Observation of pain control in patients with bisphosphonate-induced osteonecrosis using low level laser therapy: preliminary results *Photomed. Laser Surg.* **29** 447–52

Romeo U, Del V A, Capocci M, Maggiore C and Ripari M 2010 The low level laser therapy in the management of neurological burning mouth syndrome. A pilot study *Ann. Stomatol.* **1** 14–8

Rosenthal D I, Lewin J S and Eisbruch A 2006 Prevention and treatment of dysphagia and aspiration after chemoradiation for head and neck cancer *J. Clin. Oncol.* **24** 2636–43

Russi E G *et al* 2012 Swallowing dysfunction in head and neck cancer patients treated by radiotherapy: review and recommendations of the supportive task group of the Italian Association of Radiation Oncology *Cancer Treat. Rev.* **38** 1033–49

Russi E G, Raber-Durlacher J E and Sonis S T 2014 Local and systemic pathogenesis and consequences of regimen-induced inflammatory responses in patients with head and neck cancer receiving chemoradiation *Mediators Inflammation* **2014** 518261

Saleh J, Figueiredo M A, Cherubini K, Braga-Filho A and Salum F G 2014 Effect of low-level laser therapy on radiotherapy-induced hyposalivation and xerostomia: a pilot study *Photomed. Laser Surg.* **32** 546–52

Schaffer M, Bonel H, Sroka R, Schaffer P M, Busch M, Reiser M and Duhmke E 2000 Effects of 780 nm diode laser irradiation on blood microcirculation: preliminary findings on time-dependent T1-weighted contrast-enhanced magnetic resonance imaging (MRI) *J. Photochem. Photobiol.* B**54** *55–60*

Schaffer M, Sroka R, Fuchs C, Schrader-Reichardt U, Schaffer P M, Busch M and Duhmke E 1997 Biomodulative effects induced by 805 nm laser light irradiation of normal and tumor cells *J. Photochem. Photobiol.* B**40** *253–7*

Schartinger V H, Galvan O, Riechelmann H and Dudas J 2012 Differential responses of fibroblasts, non-neoplastic epithelial cells, and oral carcinoma cells to low-level laser therapy *Support. Care Cancer* **20** 523–9

Schuurhuis J M, Stokman M A, Witjes M J, Dijkstra P U, Vissink A and Spijkervet F K 2015 Evidence supporting pre-radiation elimination of oral foci of infection in head and neck cancer patients to prevent oral sequelae. A systematic review *Oral Oncol.* **51** 212–20

Scoletta M, Arduino P G, Reggio L, Dalmasso P and Mozzati M 2010 Effect of low-level laser irradiation on bisphosphonate-induced osteonecrosis of the jaws: preliminary results of a prospective study *Photomed. Laser Surg.* **28** 179–84

Shabbir M, Ryten M, Thompson C, Mikhailidis D and Burnstock G 2008 Purinergic receptor-mediated effects of ATP in high-grade bladder cancer *BJU Int.* **101** 106–112

Shiboski C H, Hodgson T A, Ship J A and Schiodt M 2007 Management of salivary hypofunction during and after radiotherapy *Oral Surg. Oral Med. Oral Pathol. Oral Radiol. Endod.* **103** S66–19

Siegel P M and Massague J 2003 Cytostatic and apoptotic actions of TGF-β in homeostasis and cancer *Nat. Rev. Cancer* **3** 807–21

Silveira P C, da Silva L A, Pinho C A, De Souza P S, Ronsani M M, Scheffer D L and Pinho R A 2013 Effects of low-level laser therapy (GaAs) in an animal model of muscular damage induced by trauma *Lasers Med. Sci.* **28** 431–6

Simoes A *et al* 2008 Effect of defocused infrared diode laser on salivary flow rate and some salivary parameters of rats *Clin. Oral Investig.* **12** 25–30

Simoes A, de Campos L, de Souza D N, de Matos J A, Freitas P M and Nicolau J 2010 Laser phototherapy as topical prophylaxis against radiation-induced xerostomia *Photomed. Laser Surg.* **28** 357–63

Simpson D R, Mell L K and Cohen E E 2015 Targeting the PI3K/AKT/mTOR pathway in squamous cell carcinoma of the head and neck *Oral Oncol.* **51** 291–8

Smith B G and Lewin J 2010 Lymphedema management in head and neck cancer *Curr. Opin. Otolaryngol. Head Neck Surg.* **18** 153–8

Smoot B, Chiavola-Larson L, Lee J, Manibusan H and Allen D D 2015 Effect of low-level laser therapy on pain and swelling in women with breast cancer-related lymphedema: a systematic review and meta-analysis *J. Cancer Survivorship* **9** 287–304

Sommer A P, Pinheiro A L, Mester A R, Franke R P and Whelan H T 2001 Biostimulatory windows in low-intensity laser activation: lasers, scanners, and NASA's light-emitting diode array system *J. Clin. Laser Med. Surg.* **19** 29–33

Song S, Zhou F and Chen W R 2012 Low-level laser therapy regulates microglial function through src-mediated signaling pathways: implications for neurodegenerative diseases *J. Neuroinflammation* **9** 219

Sonis S T 2004 A biological approach to mucositis. *J. Support. Oncol.* **2** 21–32 PMID: 15330370

Sonis S T, Hashemi S, Epstein J B, Nair R G and Raber-Durlacher J E 2016 Could the biological robustness of low level laser therapy (photobiomodulation) impact its use in the management of mucositis in head and neck cancer patients *Oral Oncol.* **54** 7–14

Sperandio F F, Giudice F S, Correa L, Pinto D S Jr, Hamblin M R and de Sousa S C 2013 Low-level laser therapy can produce increased aggressiveness of dysplastic and oral cancer cell lines by modulation of Akt/mTOR signaling pathway *J. Biophotonics* **6** 839

Sroka R, Schaffer M, Fuchs C, Pongratz T, Schrader-Reichard U, Busch M, Schaffer PM, Duhmke E and Baumgartner R 1999 Effects on the mitosis of normal and tumor cells induced by light treatment of different wavelengths *Lasers Surg. Med.* **25** 263–71

Takeda Y 1988 Irradiation effect of low-energy laser on rat submandibular salivary gland *J. Oral Pathol* **17** 91–4

Teguh D N *et al* 2008 Trismus in patients with oropharyngeal cancer: relationship with dose in structures of mastication apparatus *Head Neck* **30** 622–30

Tsai S R, Yin R, Huang Y Y, Sheu B C, Lee S C and Hamblin M R 2015 Low-level light therapy potentiates NPe6-mediated photodynamic therapy in a human osteosarcoma cell line via increased ATP *Photodiagnosis Photodyn. Ther.* **12** 123–30

van der Molen L *et al* 2012 Pre- and posttreatment voice and speech outcomes in patients with advanced head and neck cancer treated with chemoradiotherapy: expert listeners' and patient's perception *J. Voice* **26** 664–33

van der Molen L *et al* 2013 Dysphagia and trismus after concomitant chemo-intensity-modulated radiation therapy (chemo-IMRT) in advanced head and neck cancer; dose-effect relationships for swallowing and mastication structures *Radiother. Oncol.* **106** 364–9

van der Molen L, van Rossum M A, Burkhead L M, Smeele L E and Hilgers F J 2009 Functional outcomes and rehabilitation strategies in patients treated with chemoradiotherapy for advanced head and neck cancer: a systematic review *Eur. Arch. Otorhinolaryngol.* **266** 889–900

van der Molen L, van Rossum M A, Burkhead L M, Smeele L E, Rasch C R and Hilgers F J 2011 A randomized preventive rehabilitation trial in advanced head and neck cancer patients treated with chemoradiotherapy: feasibility, compliance, and short-term effects *Dysphagia* **26** 155–70

van der Molen L, van Rossum M A, Jacobi I, van Son R J, Smeele L E, Rasch C R and Hilgers F J 2012 Pre- and posttreatment voice and speech outcomes in patients with advanced head and neck cancer treated with chemoradiotherapy: expert listeners' and patient's perception *J. Voice.* **26** 664

Verdonck-de Leeuw I M *et al* 2014 The course of health-related quality of life in head and neck cancer patients treated with chemoradiation: a prospective cohort study *Radiother. Oncol.* **110** 422–8

Vescovi P *et al* 2015 Tooth extractions in high-risk patients under bisphosphonate therapy and previously affected with osteonecrosis of the jaws: surgical protocol supported by low-level laser therapy *J. Craniofacial Surg.* **26** 696–9

Vescovi P, Merigo E, Meleti M, Manfredi M, Fornaini C and Nammour S 2012 Surgical approach and laser applications in BRONJ osteoporotic and cancer patients *J. Osteoporos.* **2012** 585434

Vidovic J D *et al* 2010 Effects of low-level laser treatment on mouth dryness *Coll. Antropol* **34** 1039–43 PMID: 20977100

Vissink A *et al* 2010 Clinical management of salivary gland hypofunction and xerostomia in head-and-neck cancer patients: successes and barriers *Int. J. Radiat. Oncol. Biol. Phys.* **78** 983–91

Vissink A, Jansma J, Spijkervet F K, Burlage F R and Coppes R P 2003 Oral sequelae of head and neck radiotherapy *Crit. Rev. Oral Biol. Med.* **14** 199–212

Vissink A, van Luijk P, Langendijk J A and Coppes R P 2015 Current ideas to reduce or salvage radiation damage to salivary glands *Oral Dis.* **21** e1–10

Vissink A, van Luijk P, Langendijk J and Coppes R 2014 Current ideas to reduce or salvage radiation damage to salivary glands *Oral Dis.* **21** e1–e10

Wang CJ, Huang E Y, Hsu H C, Chen H C, Fang F M and Hsiung C Y 2005 The degree and time-course assessment of radiation-induced trismus occurring after radiotherapy for nasopharyngeal cancer *Laryngoscope* **115** 1458–60

Watters A L, Epstein J B and Agulnik M 2011 Oral complications of targeted cancer therapies: a narrative literature review *Oral Oncol.* **47** 441–8

Werneck C E, Pinheiro A L, Pacheco M T, Soares C P and de Castro J L 2005 Laser light is capable of inducing proliferation of carcinoma cells in culture: a spectroscopic *in vitro* study *Photomed. Laser Surg.* **23** 300–3

Westbury C B and Yarnold J R 2012 Radiation fibrosis—current clinical and therapeutic perspectives *Clin. Oncol.* **24** 657–72

Wigg J and Lee N 2014 Redefining essential care in lymphoedema *Br. J. Community Nurs.* **S20** s2 s4–7

Worthington H V, Clarkson J E, Bryan G, Furness S, Glenny A M, Littlewood A, McCabe M G, Meyer S and Khalid T 2011 Interventions for preventing oral mucositis for patients with cancer receiving treatment *Cochrane Database Syst. Rev.* **2011** CD000978

Yamashita H *et al* 2006 Relation between acute and late irradiation impairment of four basic tastes and irradiated tongue volume in patients with head-and-neck cancer *Int. J. Radiat. Oncol. Biol. Phys.* **66** 1422–9

Zecha J A E M *et al* 2016 Low level laser therapy/photobiomodulation in the management of side effects of chemoradiation therapy in head and neck cancer. Part 1: Mechanisms of action, dosimetric, and safety considerations *Support. Care Cancer* at press

Zecha J A E M *et al* 2016 Low level laser therapy/photobiomodulation in the management of side effects of chemoradiation therapy in head and neck cancer. Part 2: Proposed applications and treatment protocols *Support. Care Cancer* at press

www.ingramcontent.com/pod-product-compliance
Lightning Source LLC
LaVergne TN
LVHW080600210926
848485LV00003B/86
9781643278858